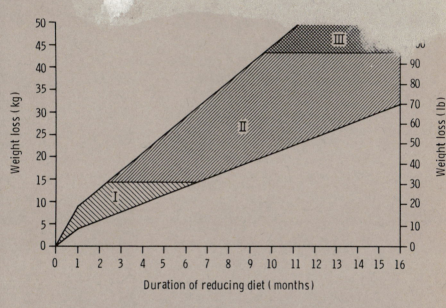

Fig. 2.1 The optimum rate of weight loss is 2 kg (4 lb) per week for the first 4 weeks, and 1 kg (2 lb) per week thereafter, but rates of weight loss not less than half this rate are acceptable. The figure shows the length of treatment (months) required to obtain a given weight loss in patients with rates of weight loss between these limits. The shading indicates the amount of weight a person with grade I, II or III obesity would need to lose in order to attain a W/H^2 of 25 (*see* Fig 1.3 for explanation of grades of obesity and *see also* page 12)

Treat Obesity Seriously

Treat Obesity Seriously
A CLINICAL MANUAL

J. S. Garrow MD, PhD, FRCP

Head, Nutrition Research Group, Clinical Research Centre;
Honorary Consultant Physician, Northwick Park Hospital, Harrow

CHURCHILL LIVINGSTONE
EDINBURGH LONDON MELBOURNE AND NEW YORK 1981

CHURCHILL LIVINGSTONE
Medical Division of Longman Group Limited

Distributed in the United States of America by Churchill
Livingstone Inc., 19 West 44th Street, New York, N.Y.
10036, and by associated companies, branches and
representatives throughout the world.

© Longman Group Limited 1981

ISBN 0 443 02306 9

British Library Cataloguing in Publication Data
Garrow, J. S.
    Treat obesity seriously.
    1. Obesity
    I. Title
    616.398   RC628

Library of Congress Catalog Card Number 81-67466

Printed in Great Britain by William Clowes (Beccles)
Limited, Beccles and London

Preface

In 1970, after many years of planning, Northwick Park Hospital and Clinical Research Centre opened to receive patients. This is a unique enterprise in clinical research: the combination of a 600-bed District General Hospital for the London Borough of Harrow with the 187-bed Clinical Research Centre, which provides excellent facilities for detailed clinical investigation of conditions which commonly occur in a hospital population.

Since the Clinical Research Centre opened I have seen about 2000 patients referred by their family doctors for advice about management of obesity. Most of these patients were given dietary advice as outpatients, but some 10 per cent were admitted to the metabolic wards for measurements of body composition and energy metabolism. That aspect of the work of our research group has been reviewed in *Energy Balance and Obesity in Man* — a monograph intended mainly for research workers in this field.

Treat Obesity Seriously is a more personal book addressed to those who are concerned with the management of obesity: it is an omnibus edition of all the letters I have written to general practitioners who asked for advice about the treatment of their obese patients. Often it is not possible to pick the optimum line of treatment at the first clinic visit, but after three or four visits it is usually possible to say what realistic options are open to a given patient, and what benefits can reasonably be expected after weight loss. The book is called a clinical manual because I hope that it will be of practical help in choosing the line of treatment which will bring most benefit and least frustration to the doctor and to his patient.

Phoenix, Arizona, 1981   J.S.G.

Acknowledgements

I am very grateful to my colleagues in the Nutrition Research Group who have been particularly concerned with research on the treatment of obesity — J. Abbott, M. A. Ashwell, S. E. Blaza, M. L. Durrant, S. Gilbert, D. Halliday, S. F. Stalley, P. M. Warwick, D. W. Wilkins —and also to the Dietetic Department of Northwick Park Hospital, without whom this work could not have been done. I also thank K.J.G., D.K.G. and S.F.S. for their helpful comments on the typescript of this book.

J.S.G.

Contents

1

Introduction

'... ONE OF THE MOST IMPORTANT MEDICAL AND PUBLIC HEALTH PROBLEMS OF OUR TIME'

The report of a study group convened by the Department of Health and the Medical Research Council under the chairmanship of Professor Waterlow began with these words:

'We are unanimous in our belief that obesity is a hazard to health and a detriment to well-being. It is common enough to constitute one of the most important medical and public health problems of our time, whether we judge importance by a shorter expectation of life, increased morbidity, or cost to the community in terms of both money and anxiety.'

This report was published in 1976, and referred specifically to the United Kingdom. In 1979 the U.S. Department of Health, Education and Welfare published the proceedings of a conference, edited by G. A. Bray, entitled *Obesity in America*. This quotation was used again, with the comment that it succinctly summarised the feelings of that conference.

How is it possible for a disease like obesity to be accorded such importance by expert committees on both sides of the Atlantic? There is no problem in diagnosis: any layman can recognise it without difficulty. It does not strike suddenly, but develops gradually over years. There is little mystery about its physiological basis: obesity occurs when, and only when, energy intake exceeds energy expenditure. That statement conceals a great deal which is not known about the regulation of energy intake and expenditure, but nevertheless the statement is true, and so is the converse statement, that obesity can be treated if, and only if, energy expenditure can be made to exceed energy intake.

Obesity is a condition in which the energy stores in the body, mostly in the form of fat, are excessively large. Recently there have been great improvements in techniques for measuring the energy stores of the body, and also for studying the regulation of energy intake and expenditure. In a metabolic ward with good facilities for dietary control it is possible to reduce excessive fat stores at a predictable rate in virtually any obese patient. It is, in principle, far easier to restore to normality an obese patient than a patient with most other diseases: even the best inpatient treatment cannot reverse the pathological changes in coronary thrombosis, chronic bronchitis, stroke, arthritis, asthma, or the great majority of diseases which afflict the hospital patient.

Why, then, is obesity such an important medical and public health problem? Why is it not easily cured, or, better still, prevented? I believe that there are three reasons for the lack of progress in this direction, none of which is insurmountable.

First, it is impossible to divide people into two categories, obese and non-obese, and to make statements about one group which are not more or less applicable to the other. Obesity is not a disease which you either do, or do not, have: rather it is a continuum, like baldness, in which the diagnosis is made when some arbitrary diagnostic boundary is exceeded. This vagueness of definition makes nonsense of attempts to characterise obesity, or even to measure prevalence.

Second, the spectrum of obesity is so wide that it cannot be covered by any one class of health professional. Severe obesity is relatively rare, but life-threatening. Surgical treatment may be the best available option, but this presents formidable problems to both surgeon and anaesthetist. The untreated person will become crippled and will eventually die in respiratory failure or succumb to the metabolic complications of severe obesity. At the other end of the spectrum mild obesity is very common, and it would be absurd to consider surgical treatment of such people. Quite different skills are required to help mildly obese and severely obese people.

Third, the majority of patients, and doctors, do not treat obesity seriously. It is not that people are indifferent, and do nothing. The level of concern among doctors is indicated by the prescription of drugs promoted for the treatment of obesity: in 1973 the cost to the National Health Service of these drugs was £2.5m, and despite official guidance that these preparations were generally ineffective the bill rose to £3.5m by 1975. Concern among the public is equally strong, and fostered by many organisations some of which have a commerical interest in treating obesity. Journalists seek avidly for news of a break-through in obesity research, because they know that they have a ready audience for items on this topic. However, this is not the same as treating obesity seriously: paradoxically, the public clamour is an obstacle to progress in this direction. Official pronouncements, such as the one at the start of this section, receive massive publicity, and this provokes counter-revelations about commercial exploitation of mini-mally overweight people. Wonder-cures are successively promoted and debunked. Any line of treatment, however well-founded or nonsensical, can be shown to have some wonderful successes and some abject failures. It is not surprising that doctors and the public are confused.

The first step forward is to stop talking about 'obesity', and to define grades of obesity: only in this way is it possible to make the management appropriate to the seriousness of the complaint.

A CLASSIFICATION OF OBESITY BY SEVERITY

The classification which has been adopted for this book is based on the index W/H^2, where W is weight (kg) and H height (m), both measured in indoor clothing, without shoes.

For simplicity the same boundaries have been applied to define grades of obesity in men and women, thus:

Grade III, $W/H^2 > 40$
Grade II, W/H^2 30-40
Grade I, W/H^2 25-29.9
Grade 0, W/H^2 20-24.9

There are many possible objections to this classification. First, it is based on body weight for a given height, and there is no guarantee that overweight indicates adiposity, it might indicate heavy musculature. This point is discussed in section 3.b. Second, those readers with mathematical inclinations may well be worried by the inappropriateness of the units involved in this index: a weight divided by the square of a length seems to denote a pressure, which is difficult to relate logically to obesity. It would be easier to accept W/H^3 which implies weight divided by a volume, which is a unit of density. The only answer to this objection is that W/H^2 is empirically useful, while W/H^3 is not. Benn (1971) has made an analysis of weight-for-height indices used as a measure of adiposity: those with the form W/H made tall people appear too fat, and W/H^3 made short people appear too fat. He concludes 'Quetelet's index will probably be as good as any if one is forced to choose blindly'. It is rather satisfying that the index W/H^2, originally proposed by a 19th century Belgian astronomer (Quetelet 1871) should regain favour with the scientific community more than a hundred years after his death.

Even if the use of Quetelet's index is accepted as a measure of obesity, the choice of 25, 30 and 40 as boundaries between grades 0, I, II and III is arbitrary and can be justified only on the grounds of convenience. The reasons for choosing the range 20 – 25 as the zone associated with minimum mortality have been reviewed elsewhere (Garrow 1979a): more precisely the equivalent of the Metropolitan

Life Insurance desirable weight-for-height over the range from the minimum for 'small frame' to the maximum for 'large frame' is 19.7 – 24.9 for men, and 19.1 – 24.6 for women (James 1976). However, when the data on which the Metropolitan Life tables were constructed are critically examined (Seltzer 1966) it is clear that there is no justification for subdivision by frame size, and that the boundaries 20 – 25 will serve well enough as a 'desirable range' of weight for height for both sexes.

It has been argued (Bateson 1979) that it is 'overgenerous' to set the upper limit of the desirable range at 25, since the ideal weight is the average weight within the desirable range. There is no evidence to support the assertion that an individual is better off with an index of 22.5 than with an index of 25, and there seems little advantage in adopting a classification which would define half the people in the ideal range as overweight. It will be evident to readers of this book that it is no easy matter to provide adequate treatment for those people in whom obesity poses a real threat to health: unnecessarily to widen the definition of obesity does a disservice to everyone.

The relationship of obesity index to mortality is illustrated in Figure 1.1. Below 20 the mortality ratio tends to increase for reasons which are not well understood: it was thought that the old life insurance statistics were influenced by mortality from tuberculosis among very thin people, but recent surveys have shown a similar upturn in mortality at very low weights (Dyer et al 1975, Lew & Garfinkel 1979, Sorlie et al 1980) which cannot be explained by tuberculosis.

The range 20 – 25 is associated with minimum mortality: this is roughly the insurance 'desirable weight' range, called, for the purpose of this book, grade 0. The increase in mortality in grade I is not very

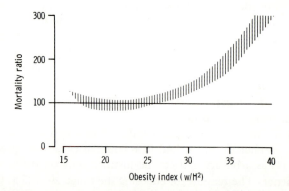

Fig. 1.1 Relation of obesity index (W/H^2) to mortality ratio. Average mortality = 100 (data of Seltzer 1966)

impressive: the importance of grade I obesity is mainly that if everyone who entered the grade I range stopped there, and progressed no further, then the clinically serious grade II and grade III problems would never occur.

Grade II represents the transition range from clinically trivial to clinically crippling obesity. At the mid-point of this range the insurance experience indicates that the mortality is roughly double that of people in the desirable weight range, and in the upper part of the range insurance statistics become unreliable because such people have great difficulty in obtaining insurance.

Grade III obesity is virtually incompatible with normal employment. There are a few young people who manage a normal job at this degree of obesity, but they certainly do not have normal exercise tolerance, and employers are aware that such people have a poor health record.

The distribution of W/H^2 values in subsets of the population in the catchment area of Northwick Park Hospital is shown in Figure 1.2: these distributions are discussed in greater detail in the chapters on the management of the various grades of obesity. The data for employed

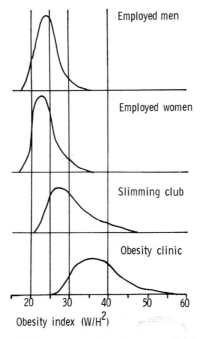

Fig. 1.2 Distribution of W/H^2 among employed men, employed women, members of a slimming club, and patients attending a hospital obesity clinic in Harrow, England

men and women come from the Northwick Park Heart Study, by courtesy of Dr. T. W. Meade. The data for slimming club members comes from the report of Seddon et al (1981): similar values can be obtained by analysis of the data of Ashwell and Garrow (1975). The obesity clinic data are based on a personal series of National Health Service patients, referred to the obesity clinic at Northwick Park Hospital by general practitioners for treatment of obesity. At the time of writing there has been no survey of the weight and height of a national representative sample of the British population, but such a survey is being undertaken by the Department of Health. It is obvious from Figure 1.2 that the distribution for W/H^2 among the whole population of men and women must be rather wider than that shown for employed men and women: those who are very thin or very fat are unlikely to be employed, and the overweight section of the population are, of course, over-represented in the slimming club membership, and even more so among patients attending the obesity clinic.

To simplify the process of classifying a given patient by obesity grade a diagram is given in Figure 1.3 in which the boundaries are indicated, and weight and height are given in both metric and imperial units. It is often useful to show a diagram of this sort to obese patients,

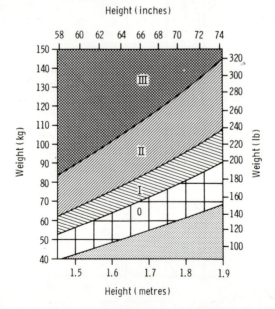

Fig. 1.3 Relation of weight to height defining the desirable range (0), and grades I, II and III obesity, marked by the boundaries $W/H^2 = 25$–29.9, 30–40, and over 40 respectively *(for easy reference this illustration is repeated on front and back end papers)*

so the individual can see how his or her own weight compares with the desirable range for height.

The format of this book: a clinical manual

This book is intended to provide guidance on how to treat obese patients. There are innumerable slimmers' books available on every bookstall exhorting fat people to adopt a diet high in this, or low in that, or to exercise more, or to forget about the whole problem. Any of these conflicting pieces of advice may be appropriate for some people, but none is effective for most, as evidenced by the continuing problem of obesity. The hospital specialist, general practitioner, dietitian or slimming club leader is constantly confronted by obese people needing help, and it is necessary to work out a plan appropriate for that particular person. It is also necessary to understand the scientific basis for the plan you recommend, and the benefits which the patient may reasonably expect in return for the inconvenience of following your advice: no sensible person will invest this effort unless he or she is convinced that the returns justify it. Astwood (1962) quotes a patient who put this point to his physician in 1825 in the following words:

'Sir, I have followed your prescription as if my life depended upon it, and I have ascertained that during this month I have lost 3 pounds or a little more. But in order to reach this result I have been obliged to do such violence to all my tastes and all my habits — in a word I have suffered so much — that while giving you my best thanks for your kind directions, I renounce the advantages of them and throw myself for the future entirely into the hands of Providence'.

Chapter 2 of this book reviews the disadvantages associated with obesity, the extent to which these are reversible by weight loss, and the effort required from both patient and therapist to achieve this weight loss. Unless both parties are convinced that the enterprise is worth undertaking it is bound to fail.

Chapter 3 reviews the scientific basis for the advice given in subsequent chapters: obesity is a disorder of energy balance, and the aim of treatment is to create a negative energy balance of degree appropriate to the degree of obesity. However there are many charlatans offering false hopes of easy weight loss, and both patient and therapist need to know why these claims cannot be true.

The remaining chapters consider the problems posed by different grades and types of obesity and indicate how an effective line of treatment may be found which does the minimum of violence to the tastes and habits of the patients, and which places demands on the therapist which are not unreasonable in the context of a National Health Service.

2

Assess priorities

The correct assessment of priorities is the key to successful management of obesity. This statement could be made about many other types of achievement: for example, the ability to play a musical instrument. Most people who at some time have tried to play no longer do so — if asked they would probably say that they 'had to give it up'. This means that their lifestyle was such that other activities had a higher priority for their available time, money and interest. However the successful concert soloist, who may have had similar circumstances, did not give up, because the pursuit of musical excellence was given a higher priority than the other activities.

A similar argument can be made with even greater force about the management of obesity. Musical virtuosity requires talent as well as determination and sound guidance, but weight loss requires no special talent, only determination and sound guidance.

It was pointed out in Chapter 1 that the different grades of obesity present different problems both to the patient and to the therapist. In order to assign priorities correctly it is necessary to judge how much effort is required to achieve a certain weight loss, and to balance this cost against the potential benefit which the patient may expect to gain. It is the job of the therapist to try to present this analysis fairly to the patient, who must then choose either to accept that the investment is sound, or else to reject it and give up or go elsewhere. It is hopeless to embark on the treatment of an obese patient without clear and realistic ideas about goals which can be achieved, and the contribution which is required from both patient and therapist. Unfortunately the obese patient is an easy prey for those who offer quick cures which do not fulfil their promises, but the honest and competent therapist has nothing to fear: in the long term the results speak for themselves.

ATTITUDES IN PATIENT AND THERAPIST

The attitude of obese patients, and of people offering treatment for obesity, shows a wide range of variation on three key issues: the benefits to be derived from weight loss, the extent to which the responsibility for maintaining treatment rests with the patient, and the demands the patient is entitled to make on the therapist.

The patient's expectation of benefit may be almost zero: some present for treatment already resigned to the hopelessness of the situation, and merely want a doctor to confirm that there is no point in attempting the impossible feat of weight loss. At the other extreme patients may be unduly optimistic on the strength of a newspaper report of a new wonder cure. Concerning the responsibility for maintaining treatment, and the rights and duties of patient and therapist respectively, there is also a wide range of opinion among patients. To some it is obvious that the cure ultimately lies in their own hands, they apologise for troubling the doctor at all, but hope that of his charity he may throw them some crumb of comfort or advice. To others it is equally obvious that the onus lies firmly with the doctor to effect a cure: if it had been a matter with which they could cope themselves they would not have wasted time consulting the doctor at all.

An equally wide spread of opinion can be found among therapists on these same issues. Some believe that it is virtually a waste of time to try to treat obesity since the results are so poor: 'most obese persons will not stay in treatment for obesity. Of those who stay in treatment, most will not lose weight, and of those who lose weight most will regain it' (Stunkard 1972). When the expected failure comes it is clearly the fault of the patient: 'we categorically accuse each subject of dietary errors whenever they fail to equal at least 85% of prediction' of weight loss (Jolliffe and Alpert 1951). If the hapless patient then fails to return at the next appointment this is final evidence of depravity: all claim to sympathy is forfeited.

Some therapists take a rather more kindly view of the patient's problem, or a less exalted view of the value of the therapist's time: perhaps helping an obese patient to avoid the penalties of obesity is no more difficult to justify than managing any other disability. Some even think that treatment failure may reflect on the therapist, and go to great lengths to be helpful. 'The therapist is available by telephone at all times, in order to guard against any failure by the patient which might adversely affect his expectation of success' (Stuart 1967). Such a deeply caring attitude is perhaps more often experienced by fee-paying patients.

BENEFITS OF WEIGHT LOSS, AND FREEDOM OF CHOICE

The tendency of overweight people to die young is well-known to life insurance actuaries (Seltzer 1966). Even more important is the observation that overweight people who were refused insurance at normal rates, but who subsequently reduced to normal weight, thereafter enjoyed normal life expectancy (Dublin 1953). The excess mortality associated with overweight bears most heavily on young people (Blair and Haines 1966): it takes some years for the effects of overweight on mortality to become evident.

The evidence cited above comes from the experience of life insurance companies, and it has been criticised on the grounds that people who take out life insurance are self-selected and not typical of the general population. However exactly the same conclusions can be drawn from the study of 750,000 men and women by the American Cancer Society (Lew and Garfinkel 1979). This large population sample was followed prospectively for 12 years, and there can be no doubt about the association of overweight with excess mortality. A 20-year prospective study of two random samples of women by Cochrane et al (1980) showed a highly significant (P<0.01) positive association between Quetelet index (W/H^2) and mortality. The evidence that significant obesity (grade II or III) shortens life is overwhelming: the only matters open to debate are the importance as a health hazard of grade I obesity, or of obesity in old age (Andres 1980). These special areas are discussed in more detail in the chapters dealing with the treatment of obesity.

Since overweight carries such severe penalties it might be supposed that there would be no problem in motivating obese patients to lose weight. Equally we might suppose that every reasonable person would wish to save money for his retirement. In practice short-term obstacles prevent the achievement of long-term objectives.

This presents an ethical problem for anyone treating obese patients. If it is agreed that it is in the interests of the patient to lose weight, and that this can reasonably be achieved by (say) six months of dieting, has the therapist done his duty by simply suggesting this course of action, or should he try to force the patient to comply with the treatment? If pension schemes relied on voluntary contributions, rather than statutory deductions from income, would pension provision be adequate? There is no doubt that people can be forced to lose weight: Scrignar (1980) describes an extraordinary situation in which overweight policemen were ordered to lose weight at the rate of at least 5 lb (2 kg) per month or be penalised by loss of leave privileges or pay. They lost weight until the order was ruled to be unconstitutional, and the sanctions were removed, when the weight was rapidly regained. Jeffery et al (1978) have reviewed publications in which patients entered into monetary contracts linked to weight loss: the stronger the contract the greater the weight loss.

Motivation for weight loss does not remain at a constant level in the obese patient. When he or she first sees the doctor enthusiasm for weight loss may verge on desperation, but this situation does not last indefinitely. At some stage resolve weakens, the diet is broken, weight is regained, and morale is destroyed. This is the sequence of events which the therapist must somehow prevent, but not by imposing a cure which is worse than the disease.

MANAGEMENT BY PROGRESS, NOT BY OBJECTIVES

The point was made in the first chapter of this book that different grades of obesity call for different modes of treatment, but every type of treatment has one factor in common: in every case we are trying to achieve a negative energy balance and consequent loss of excess fat. Techniques for studying energy balance, and the relationship of energy balance to weight change, are matters considered in the next chapter. The obese patient is probably not at all interested in such matters: he or she wants treatment which is 'successful'. If asked what 'successful' means the patient would probably reply 'the most rapid possible weight loss with minimum inconvenience' or 'getting down to ideal weight'.

The doctor should avoid the situation created by these objectives. The most rapid weight loss is achieved by total starvation, but for reasons explained later the weight loss during total starvation consists of about equal parts of fat and lean tissue. This means that if the patient achieves 'ideal weight' by total starvation it will be with a far-from-ideal body composition. Even with more sound dietary treatment 'ideal weight' may not be a worthwhile goal for some obese patients: the benefit they gain from losing the last few kilogrammes may be very poor return for the effort this requires. Everyone with experience in treating severe obesity realises that it is necessary to review the situation from time to time to see if it is more appropriate to encourage the patient to proceed to the next stage of treatment, or to settle for maintaining the progress so far made (Douglas et al 1979).

Figure 2.1 contains, I believe, the most important information presented anywhere in this book. If it were possible to have one diagram in colour, or otherwise given special prominence, this would be the diagram most deserving emphasis. The diagram shows the length of time required to lose a given amount of weight if the rate of weight loss is 2 kg/week for the first four weeks, and 1 kg/week thereafter (the upper boundary of the shaded zone) or half this rate (the lower boundary of the shaded zone). These rates of weight loss correspond to energy deficits of about 1000 kcal (4 MJ) per day, or 500 kcal (2 MJ) per day respectively.

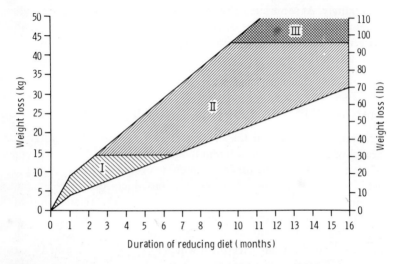

Fig. 2.1 The optimum rate of weight loss is 2 kg (4 lb) per week for the first 4 weeks, and 1 kg (2 lb) per week thereafter, but rates of weight loss not less than half this rate are acceptable. The figure shows the length of treatment (months) required to obtain a given weight loss in patients with rates of weight loss between these limits. The shading indicates the amount of weight a person with grade I, II or III obesity would need to lose in order to attain a W/H^2 of 25 (see Fig 1.3 for explanation of grades of obesity) *(for easy reference this illustration is repeated on front and back end papers)*

It is, of course, possible to manipulate rates of weight loss over short periods by tricks which are discussed in the next chapter, but these give no advantage to the patient in the long run. My definition of 'success' in treating obesity is that the patient should be losing on average 0.5–1.0 kg (1–2 lb) per week for as long as there is benefit to be derived from this weight loss. Provided that the patient also is prepared to accept this definition of success there is a good chance that treatment will indeed bring benefit to the patient. However this is not the rate of weight loss which most patients were expecting, so some will say that it is too slow, and seek some more spectacular line of treatment, possibly involving the use of amphetamines, diuretics or starvation. The disadvantages of these lines of treatment are considered in later chapters. However it is also necessary to consider another reason why patients may reject a rather slow rate of weight loss as a satisfactory line of treatment. A typical grade II obese patient with 30 kg of excess weight to lose may well look at Figure 2.1 and observe that it will take somewhere between 7 and 15 months to lose this weight and think that if the choice is between dieting for a year, or remaining fat, the latter alternative might be preferable. In some situations, especially in old patients, this may be a correct analysis. The next section concerns the disadvantages of remaining obese, which must be set against the disadvantages of having to diet.

Prolonged dieting or remaining obese: which carries the greater morbidity?

The effect of obesity on mortality has been discussed, but the obese patient may say that there is not much advantage in prolonged survival if it is only for a life made miserable by dieting. This argument would be more powerful if the life of obese people was free from morbidity, but this is not so.

Table 2.1 summarises the findings of Blair and Haines (1966) concerning the age at death of overweight people who obtained life insurance at normal premiums, having passed a medical examination. The striking feature is that the highest mortality ratio is among men 21–25 years after taking out an insurance policy, which they did at age 15–34 years. This means that the men were dying at age 36–59 years. Many obese young people, who are not unduly worried that they will not live to old age, will be much more concerned at the thought of becoming unemployable and hence a burden, rather than a support, to their young families.

Table 2.1 Mortality ratio (100 = average mortality) by weight, age at issue, and duration of policy (data of Blair and Haines 1966)

Age at issue (years)	Deviation from standard weight	Policy years				All policies
		16–20	21–25	26–30	31–34	
15–34	−23 lb or more	102	78	80	95	86
	−22 to −8 lb	77	76	91	98	86
	−7 to +7 lb	82	107	108	108	103
	+8 to +22 lb	166	131	115	94	125
	+23 lb or more	137	184	143	—	146
35–49	−23 lb or more	67	84	86	72	80
	−22 to −8 lb	79	83	77	84	80
	−7 to +7 lb	104	91	105	86	99
	+8 to +22 lb	116	117	108	119	115
	+23 lb or more	119	134	132	169	130
50–65	−23 lb or more	—	—	120	—	95
	−22 to −8 lb	97	108	102	—	100
	−7 to +7 lb	98	87	81	88	90
	+8 to +22 lb	109	102	113	—	108
	+23 lb or more	107	125	122	—	118

If the cause of death among obese people is examined closely it is clear that diseases of obese people tend to be crippling rather than killing diseases. Diabetes mellitus was 5 times more commonly the cause of death in obese men than in average-weight men (Lew and Garfinkel 1979). In obese women it was nearly 8 times more commonly the cause of death than in average-weight women. Obese diabetics do not die suddenly: these figures indicate part of the burden of disability which precedes death in obese people.

Degenerative disease of weight-bearing joints (especially back, hips and knees) and shortness of breath are important causes of disability in obese people, but they are not causes of death, so they do not appear in mortality statistics. Anyone with experience in a hospital intensive treatment unit is familiar with the difficulties in managing obese post-operative patients, but if such patients die the death is ascribed to the operation, not to the obesity.

Gallbladder disease is rather more common in obese people, but much more difficult to manage. In a thin person with abdominal pain simple clinical examination will often yield a firm diagnosis, but examination of an obese abdomen is a much less satisfactory procedure. Laparotomy is more difficult both for the surgeon and anaesthetist in obese patients, and this also contributes to the difficulty of diagnosis. Even a simple medical history is more difficult to interpret in an obese patient than a thin one: aches and pains, tiredness, shortness of breath, changes in bowel habit — these are the vague signals which alert any competent practitioner to investigate a normal-weight patient. However the identical symptoms in an obese patient are likely to be dismissed as attributable to the obesity, or the diet which the patient is supposed to be taking.

The role of obesity in hypertensive disease and ischaemic heart disease is still not clear. The association between obesity and hypertension is strong, and probably causal, but with ischaemic heart disease the relationship is only seen in men under the age of 40 years (Cook 1978).

The obese person is entitled to ask to what extent the complications of obesity can be avoided by weight loss. An attempt has been made in Table 2.2 to set out the available information on this important question.

In the case of diabetes mellitus of adult onset the improvement with weight loss is rapid and striking. Any obese person with a diabetic family history needs to take very seriously the need to reduce weight, and hence reduce the chance of developing overt diabetes. This matter is discussed more fully on page 120–123.

The effectiveness of weight reduction in reducing raised blood pressure is also well documented. Weight reduction of 10 kg is on average associated with a reduction in systolic pressure by 25.2 mm Hg, and in diastolic pressure by 15.1 mm Hg (Ramsay et al 1978).

Weight reduction will not reverse the destructive lesions in osteoarthritis, but often is more effective in giving relief from pain than any drug treatment (Dixon and Henderson 1973).

The improvement in exercise tolerance is often the first benefit noticed by obese patients who lose weight. This is in part due to purely mechanical factors, and in part to the improvement in pulmonary function which comes with weight loss (Bae et al 1976, Santesson and Nordentröm 1978).

It is reasonable to expect that weight loss would decrease the surgical and anaesthetic risks of obese patients, but no satisfactory test of this hypothesis has been published (Strauss and Wise 1978).

Gallstones certainly do not disappear with weight loss: indeed with rapid weight loss the tendency to form stones increases.

Social disability is listed among the complications of obesity in Table 2.2, because it is a common complaint among obese patients that they are socially unsuccessful. However this is difficult to investigate scientifically, and there is no convincing study to suggest that weight loss improves the situation. Psychometric testing of patients before and after massive weight loss produced by intestinal bypass indicated that their psychosocial status improved (Solow et al 1974), but Crisp and McGuinnes (1976) suggest that people are less likely to be psychoneurotic if they are allowed to remain obese.

Table 2.2 Morbidity associated with obesity, and effect of weight loss on morbidity

Complication of obesity	Effect of weight loss
Diabetes mellitus	improves greatly
Hypertension	some improvement
Osteoarthritis	usually improves
Exercise intolerance	improves greatly
Increased risk with surgery	not investigated
Gallbladder disease	no improvement
Social disability	not investigated

Willpower

It is a common journalistic cliche that the defect which causes obesity is lack of willpower. Obese patients should be able to resist the temptation to eat, but cannot do so. Willpower is conceived as an ability to suppress and discipline a natural inclination to act in a certain way.

If a pedestrian, who wanted to cross a busy road, waited for several minutes until there was a break in the traffic his action would not be ascribed to willpower, but to normal commonsense or prudence. Certainly he suppressed the inclination to step out into the road, but it is obvious that if he did so he would be likely to suffer serious injury, and his action then would be regarded as stupid or foolhardy.

When obese patients say that they know that they ought to diet, but regrettably they lack the will-power to do so, I enquire what they would do if someone were employed to follow them day and night and administer a sharp blow across the shins whenever they departed from the prescribed diet. Usually they agree that in this situation prudence would dictate that they would keep to the diet. Thus it seems that the difference between willpower and prudence lies in the immediacy of the aversive consequence. If obese people do not diet there is a high probability that they will finish up with painful legs, even if no custodian hits them on the shins, but because this consequence is more remote in time it takes an intellectual effort to recognise it as a motivating force.

The correct assessment of priorities is the key to the successful management of obesity, as I said at the beginning of this chapter. It is not only the patient, but also the therapist, who needs to make this assessment correctly. Management by progress is nonsense unless the therapist is regularly available to monitor this progress, and to provide advice and encouragement. If it is necessary to see patients at least once a month for twelve months, and if each follow-up consultation takes as little as five minutes, it means that a doctor who is treating 50 obese patients must be willing to dedicate at least one hour per week to seeing these follow-up patients. He will be able to take one new patient each week, who will require the best part of another hour for the initial assessment. Thus even with minimal patient-doctor contact for adequate supervision it will cost a practitioner 2 hours per week to manage 50 obese patients. The average general practice of 2500 patients will certainly have more patients than this who are worth treating for obesity.

Conclusions
The severity of obesity ranges from trivial to life-threatening. Obese patients should be able to obtain treatment appropriate to their degree of obesity, and should be satisfied with a rate of weight loss between 0.5 and 1 kg (1–2 lb) per week in the long term, although intially faster rates of weight loss should be attained.

The treatment strategies for different grades of obesity are described in later chapters of this book. They all involve some inconvenience both for the patient and the therapist. It is the duty of the therapist to monitor the patient's progress and to reassess from time to time the relative cost and benefit of further weight loss in this particular patient. Provided priorities are correctly assessed the treatment of obesity will bring great benefit to the health and well-being of the patient, and should provide as much satisfaction to the doctor as the treatment of any other disability.

3

The physics and physiology of obesity

THE ENERGY BALANCE EQUATION

The energy balance equation is fundamental to any rational approach to obesity. It may be simply stated thus: Change in energy stores = energy intake — energy output.

Obesity is a condition in which energy stores, mainly fat, are too large. It follows that this situation can have come about only because energy intake was too large relative to energy output. It also follows that the situation cannot be reversed unless the balance is tipped in the other direction, and somehow it is arranged that energy output exceeds energy intake.

These truths are so self-evident that it may be supposed that they hardly need stating: most people are familiar with the way in which a bank balance reflects changes in input and output, so there should be no difficulty in understanding the similar principles of energy balance. The trouble is that changes in energy stores are not necessarily reflected in similar changes in body weight. Changes in energy intake and output themselves cause changes in each other, so situations frequently arise in which the validity of the energy balance equation seems to be in doubt. It is therefore necessary to clarify the relationship between body weight and energy stores.

Energy stores and body weight

The diagram in Figure 3.1 indicates roughly the proportions of water, protein, fat, glycogen, minerals and other material in a normal adult male. Our understanding of human body composition is based largely on the chemical analysis of six adult cadavers by Mitchell et al (1945), Widdowson et al (1951), Forbes et al (1953, 1956) with additional electrolyte measurements by Forbes and Lewis (1956). This information has been supplemented by detailed chemical analysis of tissues by Dickerson and Widdowson (1960) and by many measurements using the techniques described on pages 29–34. The component about which there is least certainty is glycogen. This material is stored

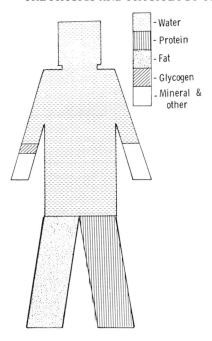

- Water
- Protein
- Fat
- Glycogen
- Mineral & other

Fig. 3.1 Diagrammatic representation of the components of body weight in a normal 70 kg adult male

mainly in muscle and liver. It it difficult to measure the total body glycogen either in living or dead subjects. In living subjects glycogen can be measured in muscle biopsies (Olsson and Saltin 1970), but since it is not uniformly distributed throughout the muscle mass there is considerable uncertainty in extrapolating from the sampled muscle to the whole body. After death muscle glycogen is the fuel for the muscular contractions known as rigor mortis, so estimations of glycogen at autopsy are not reliable indicators of the situation in the living subject.

The components of body weight which contribute to the energy stores are fat, protein and glycogen; water and mineral are irrelevant in this matter, and the component of body weight marked 'other' in Figure 3.1 is composed of material such as nucleotides and hormones which can also be neglected for purposes of calculating energy stores. The factors 4 kcal (17 kJ) per gramme for protein and glycogen, and 9 kcal (37 kJ) per gramme for fat enable us to convert the body composition shown in Figure 3.1 into energy equivalents: this calculation is set out in Table 3.1. A further complication, when trying to relate body weight to energy stores, is that body weight includes the

Table 3.1 The energy stores in the body of a normal adult male. (Values are approximate)

Component	Weight (kg)	Energy equivalent (mcal)	Energy equivalent (MJ)
Water	42.0	0	0
Protein	12.0	48	200
Fat	12.0	108	450
Glycogen	0.5	2	8
Mineral & other	3.5	0	0
Total	70.0	158	658

weight of gut contents and of urine in the bladder, although physiologically this is not material within the body.

If, when body weight changed by 5% (for example) all the components of body weight changed in similar proportion, then weight change would accurately reflect change in energy stores. This is obviously not so. During a period of total starvation body weight decreases rapidly at first, and then more slowly. The weight curve can be well described by two exponential functions (Forbes and Drenick 1979). There are at least four factors influencing this changing rate of weight loss: first, starvation is associated with ketosis, and consequent osmotic diuresis; second, during the early stage of starvation the glycogen stores become depleted, and so the water normally bound to glycogen is lost at this stage; third, there is an early loss of lean tissue, which decreases with time; fourth, there is a decrease in metabolic rate, so the energy deficit in the starving subject becomes less. With so many factors involved it is difficult to assign correct values for the relative importance of each one. The first factor, the diuresis associated with ketosis, is not essential for the early rapid phase of weight loss, since this is seen even on low-energy diets which do not cause ketosis. The effect of glycogen depletion is probably very important (Garrow 1978a), but since we have no satisfactory measure of glycogen stores this is difficult to prove. The contribution of lean tissue loss to the early rapid phase of weight loss is easily estimated from nitrogen balance measurements, (see Figure 5.9). The effect of starvation on metabolic rate and energy expenditure is discussed on pages 21 and 52.

Weight change does not reflect change in energy stores, at least in the short term, since there are situations in which water (and hence weight) is lost rapidly with concomitant loss of other tissue. It is convenient to think of the body as a mixture of lean tissue, adipose tissue, and a glycogen: water pool. Adipose tissue, as sampled by biopsy of subcutaneous fat, consists of 83% fat, 15% water and 2% protein (Garrow 1978a), so the energy value of this material should be 7550 kcal (32 MJ)/kg. Lean tissue and the glycogen:water pool both have an energy value of about 1000 kcal (4 MJ)/kg, since they contain a much higher proportion of water than adipose tissue.

Energy equivalent of weight change

Konishi and Harrison (1977) published a list of 'Body weight gain equivalents of selected foods'. The energy value of various items of food was listed, and the number of days for which this would have to be eaten in excess of requirement to produce a variety of weight gains up to 25 kg. The message was that if a person ate, for example, an apple a day too much, then over a period of 267 weeks the cumulative energy excess would be expressed as a weight gain of 25 kg. The energy value of the apple was taken to be 87 kcal, and that of weight gain 6,500 kcal/kg.

The arithmetic is correct, but the physiology is wrong. It is correct to say that anyone who gains 25 kg in 267 weeks must have had an energy intake which on average exceeded expenditure by about 80–100 kcal (400 kJ)/day, but it is not true that (as Konishi and Harrison imply) a person in energy balance who increases intake by this amout will inevitably show this weight gain. The reason why one statement is correct, and not the other, is that a change in energy intake causes a change in energy output. For this reason the energy balance equation is not so simple to apply as it seems.

During periods of weight gain energy expenditure increases, so the addition to the energy stores is less than 100% of the cumulated increase in intake. This is another way of stating a fact well known to farmers: the food conversion efficiency of livestock is always less than 100%, and there comes a stage at which it is unprofitable to increase the amount of food given to farm animals. It would be surprising if the human species, which have not been selectively bred for efficient weight gain, showed a higher efficiency than breeds which have been selected for this quality.

During periods of weight loss metabolic rate falls, so the rate of weight loss is less than might be expected for the reduction in energy intake. This decrease in metabolic rate is more than could be accounted for by loss of lean tissue during the period of dietary restriction. Figure 3.2 shows the resting metabolic rate among 103 obese patients at the start of a period of dietary restriction on the horizontal axis, and three weeks later on the vertical axis. Although the loss of lean tissue during this period was at most 3 kg, or about 5% of lean body mass, the decrease in metabolic rate is about 15%.

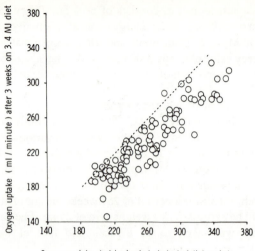

Fig. 3.2 Resting metabolic rate among 103 patients on admission to a metabolic ward, and after 3 weeks on a diet supplying 800 kcal (3.4 MJ) daily. Mean weight loss was about 5 kg

The energy equivalent of weight loss is also affected by the rate of weight loss. This is illustrated in Figure 3.3, which is based on energy balance studies on 104 obese patients (Garrow 1980). Energy deficit was calculated by measurement of energy intake and expenditure (Garrow et al 1978). At rates of weight loss below 1 kg/week the weight lost had an energy value of near to 7000 kcal (29 MJ)/kg: that is the energy value expected for adipose tissue. At rates of weight loss over 3 kg/week the weight lost shows a value of only about 4000 kcal (17 MJ)/kg: this is the value to be expected from a mixture of half adipose tissue and half lean tissue. The fact that lean tissue was being lost with the larger energy deficit was confirmed by nitrogen balance studies (Garrow 1980).

It will be evident from the foregoing discussion that, while it is true that energy excess and deficit cause weight gain and loss respectively, there are many factors which, in the short term, affect the amount of weight gained or lost for a given energy imbalance. These short-term effects are important, because they may destroy faith in the validity of the energy balance equation. The most striking example which appears to contradict the laws of thermodynamics occurs in the obese patient who has starved, or adopted a totally carbohydrate-free diet, and thus lost weight very rapidly at the expense of stripping the glycogen:water pool. Having lost about 4 kg in a week or so this patient may now eat a low-energy diet with some carbohydrate and be

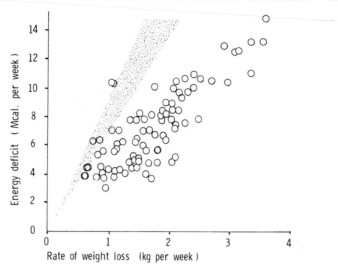

Fig. 3.3 Rate of weight loss and energy deficit among 104 obese patients on a diet supplying 800 kcal (3.4 MJ) daily for 3 weeks. The stippled area indicates the zone in which the energy equivalent of weight loss corresponds to that of adipose tissue

appalled to observe weight gain over the next day or two. Such patients are often referred to hospital with a request that their metabolism be investigated, because they have been observed to gain weight on a diet supplying, say, 1000 kcal (4.2 MJ). The truth is that on the 1000 kcal diet their energy stores were decreasing, but the weight loss which would normally have indicated this situation was masked by the increase in water (and hence weight) associated with some repletion of the glycogen stores.

In the long term, however, weight change must provide a fairly reliable indicator of the state of energy balance. The weight fluctuations attributable to changes in glycogen rarely exceed 4 kg.

Long-term regulation of body weight in man

It is commonly supposed that normal members of all species, including man, maintain a fairly constant weight in the desirable range during adult life. Certainly the laboratory rat, fed on laboratory chow, follows a predictable weight curve, and if the energy concentration of the chow is altered by adding either fat or an inert filler to the food the rats will in time compensate by eating less, or more, to achieve the same energy intake as they had before (Adolph 1947). If lesions are made in the ventromedial hypothalamic nucleus of such rats they will overeat and become obese (Kennedy 1950).

This indicates that there are centres in the hypothalamus which sense energy balance in some way which is not well understood. In the absence of any distracting factors these centres enable body weight and energy stores to be regulated. However, even in the laboratory rat, the control system is rather easily upset: if the rat is offered, not just laboratory chow, but a variety of foods available to most people in affluent countries, it will over-eat and become obese. Certainly domestic pets are liable to become obese if they are offered enough palatable food.

Opinions differ about the ability of human subjects to maintain a constant weight throughout adult life. Several distinguished nutritionists have drawn attention to the remarkable stability of their own body weight over many years (Fox 1973, Davidson et al 1979): Dr Passmore had a tail-coat made for him fourty-four years ago and it still fits him, so his energy stores cannot have changed as much as 25,000 kcal (100 MJ) in 16,000 days. This implies an accuracy of energy balance of better than 2 kcal (8 kJ) per day, or less than that 0.1% difference between intake and output.

However it is nonsense to suggest that this accuracy of regulation occurs with most people. Both life insurance data (Donald 1973) and population surveys (Gordon and Kannel 1973) show that the average weight of a population drifts upwards with time. For example the mean weight of men aged 29–39 at entry to the Framingham study was 169.1 lb (76.9 kg), and with successive examinations it increased so 12 years later the mean weight was 175.7 lb (79.9 kg). Moreover, this change of 3 kg in 12 years is small compared with the fluctuations in weight shown by most individuals: the average difference between maximum and minimum weight during the first 18 years of the Framingham study was 10 kg for both men and women (Gordon and Kannel 1973). This observation is confirmed by other surveys. Miall and Chinn (1973) conducted a survey in South Wales in connection with the aetiology of hypertension, and a large sample of men and women were examined in 1956, 1960, 1964 and 1971. Among other measurements weight was recorded. Examination of these data show that the weight of individuals changes from one examination to the next in an unpredictable manner. It is not possible to distinguish groups with particularly stable, or unstable, weight. The magnitude of the change from one examination to the next is not significantly different among those who are of normal weight compared with those who are overweight. The weight change cannot be due to serious illness, because if only those people who were present at all four examinations, and only the differences between the 1960 and 1964 weights are considered, the fluctuations in weight are still obvious (Garrow 1974).

It can, of course, be argued that if the average person regulates body weight within a range of 10 kg throughout adult life this still represents good regulation. For practical purposes it is probably good enough: a person in the grade O range at a weight of 70 kg is unlikely to come to harm from obesity at any weight between 65 and 75 kg. It is more important to enquire what has gone wrong when an individual fails to keep within the 10 kg limit and strays into the clinically important levels of obesity.

Set points and control systems

It is outside the scope of this book to make a thorough review of the large and complex literature about the mechanisms which might regulate energy balance, but one important point must be discussed. Obviously body weight and energy stores are controlled somehow, although the tightness of control is much better in some people than in others. The existence of any control system implies some reference point from which the system is being prevented from straying. For example a thermostat may be set at a temperature, and heating or cooling devices are appropriately switched to achieve that temperature in the face of external influences. The question we must discuss is the nature of the set point so far as the regulation of body weight is concerned.

An excellent discussion of set point and regulation of body weight is given by Mrosovsky and Powley (1977). In the animal kingdom there are striking examples of programming of fat stores in relation to certain biologically important events: for example fat is laid down in preparation for long migratory flights of birds which cross oceans, or in preparation for the winter sleep of hibernating animals. Does similar programming occur in man? No less an authority than Astwood (1962) has suggested that some people are destined to become obese:

'I wish to propose that obesity is an inherited disorder and due to a genetically determined defect in an enzyme: in other words that people who are fat are born fat, and nothing much can be done about it'.

Neel (1962) has suggested that diabetes mellitus is the expression of a 'thrifty genotype', and a similar argument could be made about obesity: if some people were particularly good at storing fat this characteristic would have survival value in primitive conditions where starvation was a threat to life.

Mrosovsky and Powley (1977) are impressed by the evidence that people behave as if there is some sort of set point regulation of body weight, although they are careful to state that stability of weight is not itself evidence of a set point. The publications which they cite as evidence of this stability in man are by Hervey (1969), Sims et al (1973) and Goodner and Ogilvie (1974). Hervey (1969) did not give any evidence of stability of human body weight, but cited the example based on Dr Passmore's tail-coat (see above). Sims et al (1973) reviewed their experience in a classical study of experimental overfeeding, and noted that in experimentally produced obesity, unlike spontaneous obesity, body weight returns to normal at the end of the period of overfeeding. This is indeed interesting, but the return to normal weight is not completely accurate or effortless. In the original report (Sims et al 1968) they say:

'... the volunteers found the period of weight loss emotionally more trying. Only those who had gained weight most readily had any difficulty in reaching baseline weight within several months'.

In the figure illustrating a typical subject the period of weight gain from 50 kg to 66 kg took about 200 days and the weight loss phase of about 80 days brought the weight down from 66 kg to 53 kg.

Goodner and Ogilvie (1974) reported on 174 diabetic patients followed on average for 2 years, and reported 'the remarkable stability of body weight' despite the differences in treatment. The average weight of 41 patients on insulin was 74 kg, and during the follow-up period they showed an average weight change of 3.7% from their individual mean weight. Those not on insulin had a mean weight of 77 kg with an average 2-year weight variation about the mean weight of 4.6%. This study, therefore, like the Framingham data (Gordon and Kannel 1973) shows that in most people weight oscillates over a period of a few years. The astonishing feature of the control system which we are trying to understand is that it operates so poorly in the short term, but usually rather well over a lifetime.

One hypothesis which seems adequately to explain available data has been stated thus (Garrow 1974):

'Energy expenditure is an individual characteristic, depending partly on innate metabolic efficiency and partly on the habitual level of physical activity. Energy intake is normally determined during infancy and childhood by the amount needed to satisfy hunger and support an acceptable growth rate. In adult life intake continues generally to follow the pattern established earlier in life, modified in the short term by sensations of hunger and satiety. When energy imbalance occurs in adult life it is corrected by more or less conscious effort at a stage when the change in body weight is no longer acceptable.'

Factors affecting energy intake and expenditure are discussed on pages 43 and 49 respectively. The question dealt with here concerns the idea that long-term regulation of body weight in man is effected by conscious effort, rather than by any automatic control system. To test this theory we should ideally observe a group of normal people whose weight had been altered without their knowledge, and see if they spontaneously reverted to the original weight. There are obvious practical and ethical difficulties in mounting such an experiment: no normal person whose weight is altered by more than, say, 5 kg would be unaware of the change. A less powerful, but more practicable, design is to alter weight experimentally and then observe the recovery phase during which the subject is kept in ignorance of his weight change. The results of this experiment (Garrow and Stalley 1975) show that after an increase in weight by 6 kg in 60 days by overfeeding there was no evidence of weight loss during the next 200 days. Underfeeding experiments (Keys et al 1950, Garrow and Stalley 1977) indicate that when normal subjects, who have been on a restricted diet, are given access to adlibitum food they tend to increase in weight beyond the original baseline value.

The weight chart shown in Figure 5.2 (page 86) tends to support the view that the 'set point' for the weight of an individual is some function of that person's attitude to obesity, rather than of an internal reference signal determined by hypothalamic centres or hormonal activity. In this person, during the first five years from 1972–76, weight oscillated around 90 kg. In early 1977, for domestic reasons, she ceased to believe that her weight could be controlled by dieting, and weight stability was not regained until at about 100 kg her weight again became unacceptable.

It may be that Dr Passmore's tail-coat is not evidence of a physiological set point, it is itself the set-point: suppose one day he found it did not fit, would he not then take the necessary action to return his weight to its accustomed value?

This discussion of the nature of the set point for body weight is unlikely ever to produce a definitive answer, but it is not a pointless academic quibble. If, as I suggest, a major factor in the control of body weight in both lean and obese people concerns their attitude to obesity this is good news from the therapeutic standpoint. If Astwood (1962) is correct, and obesity is the result of an inborn error, then there is not much we can do to correct the hypothetical and unidentified enzyme defect. However, if we go about it in an intelligent and determined way, there is some hope of modifying attitudes which are demonstrably unsound.

'OVERWEIGHT' AND 'OBESITY'

Obesity is a condition in which there is an excess of body fat, but in this book excess weight is used as a measure of obesity. The point is often made that the excess weight may be muscle (Parnell 1977). The objection is theoretically correct: indeed the classic work of

Behnke et al (1942) was stimulated by the rejection by the U.S. Navy of some national ranking football players on the grounds that they were overweight. It was obvious that these very fit young men were muscular rather than obese, as Behnke was able to show by methods described in the next section.

The theoretical weakness of using weight-for-height as a measure of obesity is more than counterbalanced by the practical advantages, of which the greatest is convenience. There are no easy methods for measuring body fat, or change in body fat, with anything like the accuracy with which weight, or change in weight, can be measured. The method which comes closest to meeting this requirement is by the estimation of skinfold thickness. Durnin and Womersley (1974) have published tables from which the sum of skinfold thickness at biceps, triceps, suprailiac and subscapular sites can be used to estimate percentage fat in the body. The estimates of fat from skinfold measurement were checked against measurements of density (see page 31) and the error was less than 3.5% of body weight in two-thirds of women studied, and less than 5% in two-thirds of the men (Womersley and Durnin 1977). This means that if a man changed in fat content by 5 kg it is likely, but not certain, that the measurement of skinfolds would indicate the direction of the change. By comparison, it is very unlikely that a change in weight would not correctly indicate a change of 5 kg in fat content, and the measurement of weight is far easier and requires minimal skill in the observer. It is possible to use only the triceps skinfold as a measure of obesity (Selzer and Mayer 1965): this makes the measurement less inconvenient at the cost of increasing its inaccuracy.

The other reason why it is justifiable to classify obesity by overweight is that important misclassifications will rarely arise. The example of the overweight football players has already been mentioned, but even champion athletes do not exceed $W/H^2 = 25$ except in those sports, such as Japanese Sumo wrestling (Nishizawa et al 1976), in which champions are obese as well as heavily muscled. A possible exception are the women shot-put, discus and javelin throwers studied by Wilmore et al (1977): with weight 80.8 kg, fat 21.8 kg and height 1.74m they had a $W/H^2 = 27$, but could hardly be called obese.

Relative weight, or the W/H^2 criterion, will tend to underestimate obesity in old people, but this is not clinically very important. Lesser et al (1971) showed that women aged 62–77 years were often in the normal range of weight-for-height but had a high percentage body fat. In practice it is very difficult to make a significant reduction in the fat content of elderly people without imposing greater hardship than that caused by the excess fat. In the words of the poet Gray: 'where ignorance is bliss, 'tis folly to be wise'.

Suppose an accurate and convenient method for measuring body fat became available tomorrow, would it immediately supplant weight-for-height as a measure of obesity? Probably not, because all our evidence to date about the disadvantages of obesity have been derived from weight-for-height data, since that is all that is available for large population samples. When we have large prospective studies from which we can assess the effects of fat (rather than weight) on mortality and morbidity we will know the relative value of the two measures. Meanwhile we must use what we have, and at present the most satisfactory measure is W/H^2.

METHODS FOR MEASURING HUMAN BODY COMPOSITIONS

The diagram in Figure 3.1 illustrates the approximate proportions of the components which make up the weight of a normal adult male. However the chemical analyses of cadavers, on which this diagram is based, show considerable variations between individuals. With growth and development the composition of tissues changes (Widdowson and Dickerson 1960): the infant has relatively more water, and in particular extracellular water, than the adult. When the body weight of an adult changes as a result of disease, or change of diet, there is not an equal percentage change in each of the body components, so the composition as well as the weight of the body changes. In the study of obesity, therefore, it is not enough to observe weight change, we need also to know the composition of the weight gained or lost.

Techniques for the measurement of body composition are of two types: balance techniques, which require continuous measurement of intake and output of energy or nitrogen throughout the study period, or else techniques such as total body density, water or potassium measurements which provide an estimate of body composition at one point in time. Balance techniques are far more laborious than single-measurement methods, but they can be used to test the accuracy of the simpler techniques.

Energy balance and nitrogen balance

The most accurate method for measuring the change in energy stores of a human subject is to make an exact measurement of energy intake and energy expenditure: the difference between the two measurements must equal the change in energy stores. The measurements of energy intake and output are tedious (see pages 34 and 39) and require that the subjects under study are virtually imprisoned. For these reasons the technique is rarely used, but it can yield valuable information. (Passmore et al 1958., Yang and van Itallie 1976, Garrow et al 1978). Suppose a patient eats exactly 1000 kcal (4.18 MJ) per day for 10 days, expends exactly 2000 kcal (8.36 MJ) per day, and during that 10 days loses 2.00 kg. We know that the energy equivalent of the 2.00 kg is 10,000 kcal (41.8 MJ), since that is the cumulative energy deficit. The energy equivalent of 2 kg of pure fat is 18000 kcal (75.2 MJ), and of 2 kg of lean tissue is 2000 kcal (8.36 MJ), so it is possible to calculate the amount of fat lost (x_e) from the formula:

$$x_e = \frac{E - W}{8}$$

where E is the energy deficit in Mcal, and W the weight loss in kg. In the example given $x_e = (10 - 2) / 8 = 1$. So of the 2 kg weight loss 1 kg was fat (equivalent to 9000 kcal) and the remaining 1 kg was lean (equivalent to 1000 kcal). If the energy deficit is expressed in MJ rather than Mcal the formula becomes:

$$x_e = \frac{(E / 4.2) - W}{8}$$

Figure 3.4 shows the result when this calculation is used to calculate the fat loss among 19 obese patients studied by Garrow et al (1979). It is evident that among those who lost 5–6 kg in weight some lost less than 2 kg fat, while others lost 3.5 kg of fat. It is possible that these

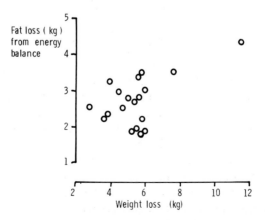

Fig. 3.4 Fat loss (calculated from energy balance) and weight loss among 19 patients studied by Garrow et al (1979)

differences are due to errors in the estimation of energy deficit, upon which the calculation of fat loss depends. We can therefore check these results against other methods for estimating fat loss.

Nitrogen balance studies follow the same plan as energy balance studies, but in this case the total nitrogen intake and output is measured. If we assume that weight loss is composed of either fat, or fat-free tissue with a nitrogen concentration of 33 gN/kg, then the weight of fat lost (x_n) can be calculated from the formula:

$$x_n = W - \frac{N}{33}$$

where N is the cumulative nitrogen deficit in gN.

Single measurement techniques: density, water, potassium

Energy balance or nitrogen balance studies can only indicate changes in body composition, they cannot yield information about the amount of fat in a person at any point in time. There are three techniques which yield estimates of body fat on a single measurement, namely density, water and potassium. There are other techniques such as skinfold measurement, which was referred to on page 00, and activation analysis (Hill et al 1978) which will not be further discussed since it is not likely to come into general use.

Behnke et al (1942) were able to show that football players were muscular, rather than obese, by demonstrating that the average density of their bodies was close to 1.10. which is roughly the density of fat-free tissue. Human fat at body temperature has a density of 0.90, so if the density (d) of the whole body is determined the percentage of fat in the body ($x\%_d$) is given by:

$$x\%_d = \frac{495}{d} - 450$$

and the weight of fat (x_d) is given by applying this percentage to the total body weight. If two such measurements are made, separated by several weeks, the change in fat stores between the two measurements should be equal to the difference between the estimates of body fat at the beginning and at the end of the study period.

It is necessary to measure the volume of the tissues of the subject with great accuracy. This has usually been done by immersing the subject in water and measuring the amount of water displaced. This has two disadvantages: first, not everyone is willing and able to immerse completely and calmly in water and remain still while a reading is taken, and second, some steps must be taken to measure the volume of air in the chest and abdomen of the submerged subject, since this will also displace water, and will make the apparent volume of the subject's tissues too large. These problems have been overcome by the use of a plethysmograph in which the subject stands in a tank of water up to neck level, and the volume of air around the head, and in the chest and abdomen, is then measured by a pneumatic principle (Garrow et al 1979).

The second single-measurement technique for estimating body fat is to measure total body water. This is done by dilution of a tracer dose of water (Halliday and Miller 1977). If we assume that fat-free tissue contains 73% water (Pace and Rathbun 1945) then the amount of fat in the body (x_w) kg can be calculated from the formula:

$$x_w = \text{Body weight} - \frac{\text{TBW}}{0.73}$$

where TBW is the total body water (kg).

The third single-measurement technique for estimating body fat depends on the assumption that fat-free tissue contains 60 mmol.K/kg in women and 66 mmol.K/kg in men. All potassium, including that in the human body, is labelled with a natural radioactive isotope ^{40}K, so each gramme of potassium emits about 3 gamma rays per second. These rays can be detected (Burch and Spiers 1953, Boddy et al 1976, Smith et al 1979) and hence total body potassium can be calculated. The fat content of the body (x_k) can now be calculated from the formula

$$x_k = \text{Body weight} - \frac{\text{TBW}}{60}$$
$$\text{(for women)}$$

$$x_k = \text{Body weight} - \frac{\text{TBW}}{66}$$
$$\text{(for men)}$$

where TBK is total body potassium (mmol).

Validation of techniques for measuring body composition

In the preceding two sections five techniques have been briefly described by which it is possible to estimate the change in fat stores in human subjects. If any one of these methods was convenient and reliable there would be no need for the others. In fact each method depends on some assumption which is not quite true, so none is totally reliable. If two methods are compared, and found to differ, it does not indicate which one is most in error, since we have no absolute standard by which to judge the accuracy of techniques for measuring body composition. However, the search for validation procedures is not hopeless, and information about relative accuracy can be obtained if many techniques are applied to the same set of subjects.

Figure 3.5 shows the estimated fat loss in the same 19 women who provided the data for Figure 3.4. In each part of the figure the fat loss estimated from energy balance is shown on the vertical axis, and on the

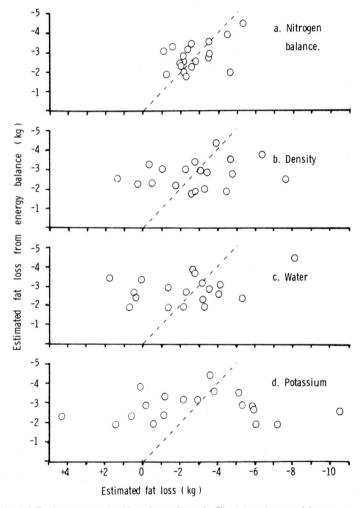

Fig. 3.5 Fat loss among the 19 patients shown in Fig 3.4: estimates of fat loss by (a) nitrogen balance, (b) change in body density, (c) change in body water, (d) change in body potassium: each compared with estimates of fat loss based on energy balance. The broken line indicates the position of points which give identical results by the pair of methods

horizontal axis the estimated fat loss from nitrogen balance, change in density, change in water, and change in potassium are shown. The broken line at 45° is where each point would lie if each of the other methods agreed perfectly with the estimate of fat loss by energy balance. It is evident that the scatter of points about this line increases with successive plots based on nitrogen balance, density, water and potassium.

There is no reason to suppose that these 19 women actually lost exactly the same amount of fat during their period of dieting so if we had a perfectly accurate method for estimating fat loss this would show some scatter between individuals. However less accurate methods would show a greater scatter, since the error in the estimation would tend to increase variability between individuals.

The five methods gave the following answers (Mean ± S.D.) for the fat lost by the 19 women studied by Garrow et al (1979): energy balance 2.77 ± 0.71, nitrogen balance 2.69 ± 1.23, density 2.83 ± 2.32, water 2.37 ± 2.38, and potassium 2.90 ± 3.54 kg. The mean values for the five methods agree which shows that the assumptions mentioned for the nitrogen, density, water and potassium content of fat-free tissue are, on average, valid. However the increasing standard deviation shows that the combined effect of measurement error, and error in assuming these values for each individual, produces a standard deviation due to error of about 1.0 kg fat with nitrogen balance, about 2.2 kg with density, about 2.3 kg with water and about 3.5 kg with potassium.

Whether or not this margin of error is acceptable depends on the purpose for which the test is being used. If, for example, two diet or drug treatments for obesity are being compared over a period of a few weeks, with fat loss of about 2 kg, then it is quite unlikely that estimates of body fat from total body potassium would detect a difference between the two groups, even if this difference existed. However if comparisons were made over longer periods, with losses of fat around 10 kg, the change in fat content then becomes large compared with the error of the measurement. The tests can also be used to show that there have not been large changes in fat content over, say, a year. If we know that fat has not changed by as much as 2 kg in a year it follows that intake and expenditure of energy must have been in balance within an average of 50 kcal (2MJ)/day (see page 30).

METHODS FOR MEASURING ENERGY INTAKE

The literature on obesity is full of failed attempts to discover what is abnormal about energy intake in obese people. Most of these projects were doomed from the outset, because the methods used for estimating energy intake were quite inadequate to detect the result which was sought. Indeed, measuring habitual food intake with accuracy is one of the most difficult tasks confronting the student of human obesity.

Dietary recall or interview

The simplest way to find out what people have been eating is to ask them to recall the nature and amount of every item of food and drink which they have consumed over the previous 24 hours. This information is entered into Food Tables such as those of Paul and Southgate (1978) and a value for energy, or any other nutrient, can be calculated. This is the technique used in many large surveys such as that of the U.S. Department of Health, Education and Welfare in 1971-. The technique rests on two assumptions:

a. that people can and will recall accurately what they have eaten over the previous day, and

b. that data from one day is reasonably representative of days in general.

Unfortunately neither assumption is valid. The report of Acheson et al (1980a) has finally shattered any illusions about the accuracy of dietary recall even among intelligent subjects working in favourable conditions. The subjects were members of the British Antarctic Survey who lived for a year at the base of Haley Bay. Every item of food had to be brought to the base by relief ship once a year, so it was very easy to check food consumption among 12 members of the expedition. For a total of 1085 man-days the subjects kept weighed records of all items of food and drink, and on 86 occasions they were asked to recall what they had just recorded for the previous 24 hours. This task is obviously much easier than that of a person who is asked to recall intake which he had not recorded, but even with this advantage the recalled intake ranged from 33–132% of the recorded intake. When the subjects were given a blank sheet of paper on which to recall their intake they underestimated on average by 33.6%, while if they were given a printed dietary questionnaire they underestimated by one 21% on average. The only reasonable conclusion from this report is that it is a waste of time for both investigators and subjects to use dietary recall data, because the results are so unreliable that it would be easier, and just as accurate, to make a guess at energy intake based on the published average values for energy requirements.

An attempt to improve on the recall procedure is the research dietary interview (Burke 1947). A trained interviewer asks about the food eaten at meals in the recent past, and if these were typical or not. More questions concern the general eating pattern, and the extent to which it is altered when eating away from home. This information is cross-checked against data on total food purchases for the week, and the amount of money spent on food. With a skilled interviewer and a cooperative subject Reed and Burke (1954) estimate that intake of specific nutrients, like protein, can be estimated with a standard deviation of about 10%, but the error for energy estimates is probably greater. However, the best any dietary interviewer can do is to find out what people believe they are eating, and it is obvious that this is sometimes far from reality. Often obese patients may be followed in the outpatient clinic for months maintaining a stable weight, and repeated dietary interviews yield estimates of intake around, say, 1000 kcal (4.2 MJ) per day. When such patients are admitted to a metabolic ward and studied under close supervision (Garrow et al 1978) it is obvious that their energy expenditure cannot be less than, say, 1600 kcal (6.7 MJ) so the outpatient dietary interview estimates must have been wrong by some 60%.

Observed eating in public places

Since people are so bad at remembering and reporting what they eat, the alternative is to observe them. Techniques which involve weighed inventories of food consumed, and which therefore cannot be done without the knowledge of the subject, are considered in the next section. It is better to observe food intake unobtrusively if possible, because the observer will then not affect the phenomenon which he is observing.

Stunkard and Kaplan (1977) review the 13 studies of eating behaviour in public places which had been published up to that time. The variables that were considered were food choice, meal duration, mouthfuls/meal, chews/mouthful, mouthfuls/minute, amount/mouthful, and amount/minute. The results indicated that obese people might choose more food, and eat it more quickly, than non-obese people, but there was not complete agreement on this. In a recent study Coll et al (1979) observed over 5000 food choices at various eating establishments, and concluded that the major influence on how much people chose to eat is where they eat, and that obesity is not a major determinant of food choice in public places.

Observation of eating at home is time-consuming and socially difficult: subjects who agree to this plan (Waxman and Stunkard 1980), and their behaviour under observation, may not give a true indication of how the average non-observed person behaves.

Weighed dietary inventories

The classical study of Widdowson (1936) on the food intake of individuals was done by getting each subject to weigh and record each item which was eaten during one week. The results showed twofold variation, not related to body weight, and were treated with some scepticism, since the scatter might represent the failure of some subjects to keep accurate records. However there is no doubt that there are very large differences in the amount of energy eaten (and used) between normal individuals, and from day to day with the same individual. The opportunity for meticulously controlled dietary inventories arises seldom: it requires subjects who accept curtailment of their liberty to go where they please, and eat what they like, without the tedium of weighing and recording every item. One opportunity arose with the British Antarctic Survey team (Acheson et al 1980a): in the nature of their job these people were forced to live in a closed community and eat from a common catering system. The average energy intake among the 12 subjects of this study ranged from 2430 kcal (10.2MJ) to 3970 (16.6 MJ) per day, and the coefficient of variation from day to day ranged from 18.2% to 42.1%.

It could be argued that polar explorers are not like ordinary people, and the curious conditions in which they live might make their eating pattern more erratic. However similar ranges of variation have been found in every other group which has been carefully studied, notably members of religious communities (van Stratum et al 1978, Groen et al 1962) and soldiers in training (Widdowson et al 1954, Edholm et al 1955, 1970). Figure 3.6 is taken from the data of Edholm et al(1970). It shows the maximum and minimum food intake per day among 55 infantry recruits during their 3 weeks of initial training. These were all fit young men, undertaking similar vigorous physical

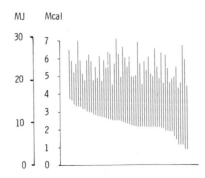

Fig. 3.6 The range of daily energy intake among 55 soldiers studied by Edholm et al (1970)

activity, and on average their energy intake matched their energy expenditure well. In an earlier study of 12 cadets over a period of 14 consective days (Edholm et al 1955) there is a similar range of variation from person to person, and from day to day.

Mesurement of energy intake by weighed dietary inventory is a good method for a captive and disciplined group of subjects. The outstanding question is: for how long must the observations be made to indicate habitual intake?

It is obvious that measurements on a single day are virtually useless, since the day-to-day variation is so great. Measurements over one week are much better: in the study by Acheson et al (1980a) the coefficient of variation from day to day was 18.2–42.1%, but from week to week was 5.9–28.9%. In the study by Edholm et al (1955) the individual intake values for each cadet are given for each of the 14 days of the study. If the intake during the first 7 days is used to predict intake during the next 7 days the average error is 261 kcal (1.1 MJ) per day, or about 8% of average intake. The conditions under which these measurements were made were near to ideal both for accuracy and for reproducibility of experimental conditions. The subjects were under military discipline and accustomed to regimentation, trained observers were employed to monitor the food intake of each cadet at every meal, and the same conditions applied to the first and second weeks of the study. We must conclude, therefore, that however intensively the eating habits of people may be studied it is impossible to predict their energy intake over a period of a week with an accuracy much better than 10%.

Laboratory studies of eating behaviour

If subjects are removed from ordinary civilian life, and fed on a diet prepared in the laboratory, it is very easy to measure energy intake: the accuracy is limited only by errors in weighing the food, in estimating plate waste, and in analysing the energy content of the food by bomb calorimetry. The problems of measurement can be still further simplified by providing a feeding machine from which the subject can obtain on demand either liquid (Hashim and van Itallie 1965, Campbell et al 1971, Pudel and Oetting 1977) or solid (Durrant and Wloch 1978) food. With liquid food it is particularly easy to alter the energy density of the food without altering the flavour or texture, and thus to test the ability of subjects to sense disguised changes in energy content (Wooley et al 1972). Studies of this sort do not pretend to measure normal food intake, since they are conducted in an abnormal setting, but they may give indications of the factors which regulate food intake. This topic is discussed on page 43.

METHODS FOR MEASURING ENERGY EXPENDITURE

Fortunately, energy expenditure is less labile than energy intake, and less likely to be affected by experimental conditions. For example a person who is in energy balance, consuming and expending 2500 kcal (10 MJ) per day, could choose one day to eat nothing, or more than twice his requirements. Energy expenditure cannot be altered at will over such a wide range: the minimum is set by basal metabolism (say 1500 kcal (6 MJ) per day), and the maximum by his capacity for sustained work — an extra 1000 kcal (4 MJ) would be about the limit for anyone who is not unusually fit. Therefore it is more justifiable to make measurements of energy expenditure over fairly short time samples and extrapolate these results to give an estimate of typical energy expenditure.

Direct calorimetry

The measurements of Atwater and Benedict (1899) were made on Mr E Osterberg, a laboratory janitor and chemical assistant. This uncomplaining man, of Swedish extraction, was sealed into a box 2.15m × 1.22m × 1.93m for periods of 4 days at a time, and the heat produced by his metabolism was removed by cold water circulating in pipes inside the chamber. From the temperature rise in the water, and the flow rate, his metabolic rate was calculated with great accuracy. However the work involved in measuring and calculating transfer was very great, so Atwater and Benedict (1905) described 'A respiration calorimeter with appliances for the direct determination of oxygen', since they were able to show a close relationship between heat production and oxygen consumption. Since that time most measurements of energy expenditure in man have been done by indirect calorimetry, that is, by measurement of oxygen uptake and carbon dioxide production, rather than by measurement of heat production.

However direct calorimetry has survived as a technique for two reasons: first, it is impossible to estimate energy expenditure in ruminant animals by indirect calorimetry, and second, because it is a more accurate technique for long-term measurements in man (Garrow 1978a). Technology has improved greatly, so modern calorimeters do not need the teams of technicians working round the clock which Benedict employed. New materials for the walls of calorimeters measure heat flow (Benzinger et al 1958, Spinnler et al 1973), heat sink calorimeters similar in principle to that of Benedict have been made more automatic (Garrow et al 1977, Dauncey et al 1978), or may take the form of a water-cooled garment surrounding the subject (Webb et al 1972). Tschegg et al (1979) describe a calorimeter in which air is cooled precisely before entering the chamber, heated by the subject as it passes through the chamber, and then heated again by a precision thermostatically controlled heater to a predetermined energy level, while the version by Brown et al (1977) is certainly the cheapest: it uses cool water from the mains supply to take a fixed rate of heat out of a small chamber, and then uses an electric heater to maintain a constant temperature.

It is beyond the scope of this book to discuss the relative merits of different types of direct calorimeter: they vary greatly in their performance and cost. Figure 3.7 illustrates the direct calorimeter at the Clinical Research Centre, Harrow. Its advantages are that it was relatively inexpensive to construct, it is acceptable to most patients for measurement periods of 26 hours, and it gives an estimate of 24 hour energy expenditure which is reproducible within about 2% under fairly standard conditions. Its main disadvantage is that it does not permit separate measurement of heat loss by evaporative, convective and radiative routes, but registers the sum of total heat loss, which, for energy balance studies, is what we require.

The chamber is similar in size to that of Atwater and Benedict (1899), and 6 m³ in volume, with walls of expanded polystyrene 20 cm thick, lined inside and outside with aluminium (P). Air is circulated by

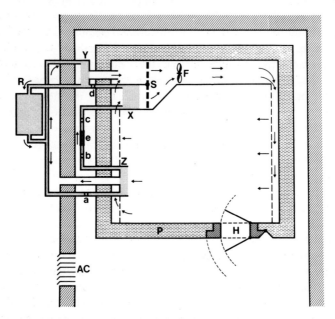

Fig. 3.7 A direct calorimeter built at the Clinical Research Centre in 1976: see text for description

a fan (F) at 3 m³/minute in a duct along the rear wall under the bed. The end walls of the chamber have false walls of perforated hardboard, so the circulating air emerges from the perforations in the right-hand wall, and passes in a laminar flow fashion across the chamber to enter the perforations in the left-hand wall. During the passage across the chamber it picks up heat from the subject. This heat is removed by a heat exchanger in the duct under the bed. The proportion of the air flow which goes through the heat exchanger is controlled by a semicircular shutter(s) driven by a servo motor. The servo motor is in turn controlled by thermistors which monitor heat flow across the walls of the chamber, and the whole system is adjusted for zero heat flow across the walls. Thus the amount of heat lost by the subject equals the amount of heat gained by the heat exchanger (X).

The heat exchanger is supplied with cold water from a refrigerated reservoir (R) in an adjacent room. This water passes in series through a reference heater (e), at which point exactly 100 watts is injected into the water, and then to the main heat exchanger. The temperature rise across the heat exchanger is in the same proportion to the temperature rise across the reference heater as the heat loss of the subject is to 100 watts. In order to supply the subject with fresh air 50 l/min of air is admitted to the chamber through a subsidiary heat exchanger (Y) and an equal amount of chamber air is removed through a twin heat exchanger (Z). Entry to the chamber is by a door containing a window and pass-through hatch (H), and the room housing the chamber is maintained at a constant temperature by an air conditioning unit (AC). Thus it is possible to observe the heat loss of a subject throughout the 24 hours, eating, sleeping, watching television, or (if desired) riding a bicycle ergometer. It is not necessary to make any assumptions about the energy equivalence of respiratory gases (see below) and the apparatus can easily be calibrated by either an electrical heat source or a butane lamp with known energy output.

Indirect calorimetry
The simplest apparatus for indirect calorimetry is that shown in Figure 3.8, which is taken from a publication by Benedict (1930). The blower (B) draws air from the helmet over the subject's head through soda-lime, which absorbs the carbon dioxide produced by the subject. The rate at which oxygen is being removed by the subject is indicated by the change in volume in the spirometer (S) and recorded on the revolving kymograph drum (K). However apparatus of this sort is very vulnerable to errors arising from leaks around the neck seal, and to changes in volume due to changes in temperature or atmospheric pressure, rather than to metabolic uptake of oxygen.

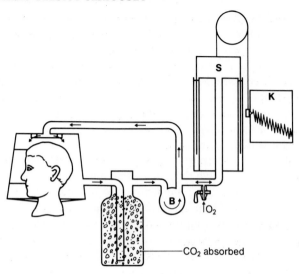

Fig. 3.8 One of the earliest ventilated hood designs, from Benedict (1930)

Modern physical gas analysers make analysis of expired air relatively simple, so it is no longer necessary to use volumetric techniques. Various types of open-circuit ventilated hood systems have been described (Ashworth and Wolff 1969; Garrow and Hawes 1972; Kinney 1980): the problems lie not in the plumbing but in the interpretation of the observed gas concentrations coming from the hood (Garrow 1978a, Johnson 1980). Open circuit respiration chambers can be made quite quickly and cheaply (Gurr et al 1979) but they present problems with the control of temperature and humidity. An ingenious 'open and shut' respiration chamber has been described for use with large animals (Blaxter et al 1972): it has the advantages of a closed circuit chamber, but saves the considerable cost of absorbing carbon dioxide by periodically venting the chamber to atmosphere and filling it with fresh air.

For subjects at work in the field portable respirometers are used which measure the volume of expired air, and either save a sample for later analysis, or, in the new 'Oxylog' devices (Humphrey and Wolff 1977) perform the analysis and calculations in a small battery-operated pack.

The activity diary
In order to obtain an estimate of the energy expenditure of subjects not confined in a calorimeter chamber it is necessary to estimate the energy

cost of individual activities, and to record the time spent in each activity. A review of a long series of such studies is given by Edholm (1977). Ideally observers should be employed to note the time spent in each activity, but alternatively the subject is required to keep a record of his own activities. It is fruitless to debate the errors involved in this method, since they will depend on the pattern of activities and the accuracy with which the record is kept. I have recorded my own exasperation when trying to remember to keep an accurate activity diary (Garrow 1978a), and evidently the irritation was felt also by subjects who were prepared to endure antarctic conditions (Acheson et al 1980b).

If it is impractical to measure the energy cost of each activity for the subjects under study, the activity diary method may be used by substituting typical energy costs for activities such as walking, sitting, standing, etc. from the extensive tables of Passmore and Durnin (1955). Since the energy cost of activities varies greatly between individuals this policy increases the error of the estimate.

Heart rate records
During strenuous physical exercise the demand for oxygen, the output of the heart, and the pulse rate all increase. There is quite a good relationship, in any one person, between heart rate and energy expenditure during exercise. Unfortunately the relationship is not nearly so close in subjects at rest, when the demand for oxygen is not driving up the heart rate. Posture and emotional factors then affect the heart rate independently of energy expenditure.

However modern electronic heart rate monitors have been extensively used to estimate energy expenditure (Warnold and Lenner 1977, Acheson et al 1980b).

FACTORS AFFECTING ENERGY INTAKE, AND ABSORPTION FROM THE GUT

About ten years ago it was thought that obesity was an 'eating disorder' (Stunkard 1972): that normal people ate normally, but obese people had some defect in the regulation of intake. It is still true that obese people have eaten more than they required, but it is by no means clear that the eating behaviour of the great majority of obese people is in any systematic way different from that of the great majority of normal-weight people. It is evident from the work reviewed on pages 35–38 that eating by 'normal' people is erratic, and obese people would have to behave very oddly indeed to produce an eating pattern which was demonstrably different from 'normal'. Schachter (1968) claimed that stimuli unrelated to requirement for food were more likely to trigger eating in obese people than in lean controls, and much behaviour therapy is based on this premise. However recent work has tended to show that although Schachter was right in saying that obese people eat for all sorts of reasons other than a need for food, this statement is equally true of most non-obese people also. Irrational eating behaviour is more obvious in obese people because their eating is more likely to come under scrutiny.

This section on factors affecting energy intake is therefore not specifically about obese people, but about people. Even if we accept that obesity is not an eating disorder we still need to learn as much as possible about the factors controlling eating, since the treatment of obesity inevitably involves trying to reduce energy intake. It is impossible to make an adequate review here of the biochemical, hormonal, nervous, behavioural and social factors which have been shown to affect eating. Readers who require a guide to this vast literature should consult the proceedings of one of the many conferences in this field: for example, *Appetite and food intake*, edited by T. Silverstone, Dahlem Konferenzen, 1976, and *Hunger, Basic mechanisms and clinical applications*, edited by D. Novin, W. Wyrwicka and G. A. Bray, Raven Press, 1976.

Hypothalamic control of energy intake

There are two regions in the hypothalamus which are of great importance in the control of feeding. Classical work, which is reviewed in the symposia mentioned above, showed that if lesions are made in the lateral part of the hypothalamus animals cease to eat and become apathetic and eventually die of starvation unless force fed. This region was therefore labelled the hunger centre. If lesions are made in the ventro-medial part of the hypothalamus animals eat voraciously and become obese, so the ventromedial nucleus was called the satiety centre. These results of experimental lesioning are still true and reproducible, but the interpretation of the results has changed greatly in the past few years. Destruction of the lateral hypothalamus causes apathy rather than anorexia, so animals with this lesion may actually eat more if they are given the stimulant drug amphetamine, although in normal animals amphetamine, reduces food intake. The work of Gold (1973) showed that the effects which had been ascribed to lesions of the ventromedial nucleus were in fact attributable to damage to nearby tracts: the nucleus itself was not concerned with the regulation of food intake.

This new research has shifted attention away from the hypothalamus towards peripheral sensors. The hypothalamus is a telephone exchange rather than a command centre: we need to know what messages it receives and where they come from. Booth (1978) has proposed a computer model of the control of human feeding in which gastric emptying rate, lipogenesis, lipolysis, hunger, satiety and eating rate interact to maintain a constant net flow of utilised energy. It is interesting that this model requires no set point for body weight (see page 25), whereas other formulations, such as that of Russek (1976) postulate a set point. When it comes to validating such mathematical models by comparing their predictions with what actually happens to people there are difficulties of two types. First, for a given set of circumstances models behave consistently, whereas people do not. This does not mean that the model is wrong, but it means that it is incomplete: there must be other factors operating which the model does not recognise. The second type of problem is that models predict hunger, appetite or satiety, and these are very difficult things to measure in man. The easiest experiment to conduct and interpret is one in which some environmental factor is manipulated and the amount the subject eats is then observed. It is generally more satisfactory to record the amount eaten than the subjects' views on what they would have eaten (Blundell 1979).

Can energy intake be perceived?

In normal life people know what they are eating because they recognise familiar food and the amount which they are accustomed to eat. However, if deprived of this information, would people still know if they had eaten more or less than normal? To answer this question Wooley et al (1972) gave obese and non-obese subjects a liquid meal, which was of the same energy content as that subject's normal meal, for a baseline period of 5–10 days. Over the next 14–10 days the subjects were given a liquid meal of similar taste and texture, but with either half or double the normal energy content. They were asked to estimate each day if the meal had been high or low in energy. Subjects recorded their estimates over a period up to the next normal meal, and were allowed to alter their judgement at any stage if they so desired. Over a series of 262 meals neither obese nor non-obese subjects showed any ability to judge correctly if they had been overfed or underfed at that meal.

This was an interesting study. If people could perceive the energy content of a meal it is hard to see why the subjects did not score significantly better than 50% correct estimates which they would achieve by change. However if people cannot perceive the energy content of a meal (as seems to be the case), yet energy intake is somehow controlled, there are three possible ways in which this could be done. First, energy intake might be controlled primarily by recognising what you are eating, so covert change in energy intake would not be detected. Second, the detection of energy intake might be unconscious, so the control system would operate, but the subject would be unable to report correctly the energy content of a meal. Third, a two-fold change in the energy content of a single meal might be too small a signal to detect, so it might require several days of overfeeding or underfeeding to bring the control system into operation. There is some experimental evidence in favour of each of these explanations: it is possible that all three are partly true.

The effect of energy density of the diet on energy intake

Hunt et al (1975) observed that obese people tend to eat a diet with a higher energy concentration than that eaten by thin people. They postulate that the rate at which energy was absorbed would be greater with the higher energy diet, since the gastric emptying would be relatively faster. Several attempts have been made to find out if people will adjust their intake of food to maintain a constant energy intake when the energy concentration in the diet is covertly altered. (Campbell et al 1971, Wooley 1971, Spiegel 1973). It is quite difficult to devise an experiment in which subjects eat a normal amount of the experimental food: the studies of Campbell et al (1971) are un-convincing because their subjects ate so little from an automatic feeding machine. However Porikos et al (1977) used an artificial sweetener to achieve a change in energy density of normal food, and their subjects ate more than enough to maintain weight. Durrant (1980) used preloads of different energy content, and tested lean and obese subjects on a feeding machine. The general conclusion from all of these experiments is that, although some subjects make some adjustment to compensate for a covert change in the energy density of food, the effect is never very impressive.

The effect of palatability on energy intake

It is obvious that people and animals will eat more of a diet which they find palatable than one which they dislike. However any food loses its attraction if it is the sole item in the diet, so it is to be expected that food intake would be greater with a varied diet than with a monotonous one. This has been demonstrated in man (Cabanac and Rabe 1976) and animals (Sclafani 1978).

An interesting theory was proposed by Cabanac and Duclaux (1970) that obese and lean people differed in their reaction to sweet taste: after a meal lean people found sweet solutions unpalatable, whereas obese people did not develop an aversion to sweet taste after a meal. This suggested that satiety aversion to sweetness was a normal part of appetite regulation which obese people lacked. However the theory is unproven, and other workers have failed to find this difference in response between lean and obese subjects (Grinker 1978).

The effect of exercise on energy intake

People engaged in hard manual labour have relatively high energy requirements, and must eat correspondingly. However Mayer has suggested that at very low levels of exercise there is a paradoxical increase in energy intake, which leads to obesity (Mayer et al 1956). The animal and human experiments supporting this conclusion have been reviewed in some detail elsewhere (Garrow 1978a): there is no evidence that if a sedentary person becomes moderately active his energy intake tends to decrease. Inactivity certainly decreases energy expenditure, so if it also increased energy intake obesity would be very common in inactive people. Of course many grossly obese people are perforce inactive, but this may as well be an effect as a cause of the obesity. If inactivity alone caused obesity this should be a major problem among paraplegic patients who were active until they were immobilised by a spinal injury, but this does not seem to be the situation (Garrow 1979b).

The effect of stress on energy intake

Stress is difficult to define, or to investigate experimentally. It is common for obese patients to say that they overeat in response to stress, or that they eat for comfort. This popular belief is reflected in the German word 'Kummerspeck' or 'worry fat' (Pudel and Oetting 1977). However Robbins and Fray (1980) in a critical review, conclude that while eating may be induced by stress it does not act to reduce that stress. This observation fits in well with the behaviour of people who have their teeth wired together to stop binge eating in response to stress: although the response to stress is prevented they experience no greater stress as a result.

Conditioned satiety

For many years there have been two great mysteries concerning the control of food intake in man:

a. How does the signal for satiety work in time to stop the meal? Whatever the signal may be — a change in blood glucose, a change in body temperature, even the taste of the food — it cannot be generated until the food has at least entered the mouth, and once in the mouth it is likely to be eaten rather than spat out. It is difficult to believe that a person who needs, say, 500 kcal (2 MJ) at a particular meal would rely on a satiety signal generated half-way through the meal to terminate it at 500 kcal, because there is no certainty that, having set up conditions which would produce satiety some time later, the second half of the meal would actually be eaten. Therefore if we believe that the signal comes from the last mouthful actually eaten, how can this operate in time to stop the next mouthful when there is probably less than a minute for the last mouthful to be analysed by the control system, whatever that may be?

b. Since the control system seems to work well in the long term, how is it possible to fool it so easily in the short term with changes in the energy density of food (see page 46)?

Both these problems may be explained on the hypothesis that satiety is a conditioned reaction: that it arises, not from the properties of the meal which we are currently eating, but from our experience of similar meals which we have eaten in the past. If our past experience is that about 500 kcal is a comfortable and satisfying amount to eat at a particular meal we will experience satiety when we think that we have eaten about 500 kcal. If some scientist has adulterated the food, so that when we think we have had 500 kcal we have in fact had more or less, this will not affect satiety until the experiment has gone on long enough for us to acquire a new set of experience about the consequences of eating the adulterated food.

The history of this important idea is given by Booth (1977). It is important from a clinical viewpoint, because it offers hope that a satiety mechanism may be susceptible to retraining. A convincing demonstration of the acquired sensory control of satiation in man was given by Booth et al (1976). They recruited university staff and students to take 100 ml of a starch drink before a sandwich lunch, with a flavoured yoghurt as dessert. Every day the lemon-flavoured starch drink looked and tasted the same, but on some days the drinks contained 5 g starch and the yoghurt was one flavour, and on other days the drink contained 65 g starch and the yoghurt was a second flavour. In time subjects came to eat less on the days when the meal started with the higher starch preload, than when it started with the smaller starch preload. So far the experiment has told us nothing about the mechanism by which this adjustment was made. The second phase of the experiment was to change all the starch drinks to an intermediate value (35 g starch) and observe the effect of the flavour of the yoghurt dessert on the amount eaten at the meal. At first, when subjects were offered the flavour of yoghurt which had previously been associated with the large starch preload they ate less yoghurt than when offered the flavour previously associated with the small preload. When the experiment was repeated with the 35 g preload several times the difference disappeared. This is as convincing evidence as possible that the subjects had come to associate a flavour with a particular state of satiety under conditions when this association was appropriate, and had continued to make the association even when there was no reason for it.

The idea that habit, experience and teaching are important influence in regulating food intake is one supported by much animal experimentation. The phenomenon of 'bait shyness' is well known: if an animal has been injured by eating poisoned food neither that animal, nor other members of the same colony, will eat food of the same flavour, even if unpoisoned food is offered. It is obvious that this learned aversion to certain types of food is necessary for survival of the species, and it is not difficult to accept that similar types of conditioning are powerful factors in determing the amount, as well as the type, of food eaten. The system breaks down when conditions change, and experience is no longer a reliable guide. In the case of human obesity it is striking that migrants from a less affluent to a more affluent culture may experience a very high incidence of obesity. Presumably it takes time to learn the appropriate intake of new and palatable foods.

Absorption of energy from the gut

Some surgical treatments of obesity are designed to reduce intestinal absorption of nutrients, particularly of energy (see pages 76 and 140). It is often suggested that some obese people must absorb the energy from food unusually efficiently, and thus have a higher intake in metabolisable energy than expected for their food intake, or alternatively that people who remain thin while eating heartily have malabsorption (Macnair 1979).

There is no evidence for this view. Loss of significant amounts of energy in faeces is rare, even in those patients who are investigated in hospital (Garrow and Wright 1980). In normal people absorption of energy is about 95% of intake, so there is little room for extra efficiency. Innumerable studies on the faeces of obese patients have failed to show that they were particularly efficient in absorbing energy, and overfed subjects do not dispose of the excess energy by reducing the proportion of energy absorbed from the gut (Norgan and Durnin 1980).

RESTING METABOLIC RATE AND THERMOGENESIS

Total energy expenditure can be measured using the techniques described on pages 39 to 43. It is convenient to consider energy expenditure in three parts: basal or resting metabolism, which is the energy required to maintain metabolic processes in the resting post-absorptive state; energy expenditure in excess of resting metabolism due to activity in skeletal muscle; and energy expenditure in excess of resting metabolism from all causes other than exercise.

The effect of exercise on energy balance is considered on pages 154–163. The following sections will discuss resting metabolic rate, and 'thermogenesis' — a term which is used to denote increase in metabolic rate above the resting level for reasons other than exercise.

The contribution of resting metabolism to total energy expenditure

The importance of resting metabolic rate in determining daily energy expenditure is usually underestimated. For example Passmore and Durnin (1955) say

'A departure of 10% above or below the normal basal level involves an error of only some 50 kcal throughout a night's sleep, which is a very small proportion of the total 24 hour energy expenditure'.

This is true, but that basal sets the level of energy cost for all other activities. This is illustrated in Table 3.2. Warwick et al (1978) made a detailed study, by both direct and indirect calorimetry of two young women who differed greatly in energy intake and expenditure. One subject, N.B., habitually ate about 2370 kcal (9.9 MJ) per day, and on direct calorimetry on three occasions she was found to have corresponding heat losses. The other subject, E.T., who was identical in age and build, was a small eater, and habitually ate about 1545 kcal (6.5 MJ) per day. The total energy expenditure of the two subjects when confined in a direct calorimeter for 24 hours was rather less than

Table 3.2 Total energy expenditure, and energy cost of particular activities in a 'large eater' (N.B.), and 'small eater' (E.T.) data of Warwick et al 1978

	N.B.	E.T.	N.B./E.T.
Total energy expenditure (kcal/day)	2142	1512	1.42
Metabolic rate (ml O_2/min)			
Lying	236	175	
	240	181	
	234	171	1.35
Sitting	238	180	
	246	180	1.34
Standing	256	179	
	258	204	1.38
Treadmill walking 5 km/h	1274	1046	
	1094	878	1.23

their habitual intake: 2142 and 1512 kcal respectively. This is to be expected, since both were usually more active when outside the calorimeter than when in it.

However the striking fact about these two young women was that the large difference between them in daily energy expenditure could not be explained on the basis of a differences in their level of activity, but on the difference in the energy cost of the same activity. Whether lying, sitting, standing or walking N.B. always had an energy expenditure about 35% greater than that of E.T. for the same activity. We can calculate that if N.B. spent the entire 24 hours at rest she would use about 1650 kcal, while E.T. would use about 1220 kcal. So of the observed 630 kcal difference between them in total energy expenditure in the direct calorimeter 430 kcal can be explained by the energy cost of resting. Furthermore the energy cost of lying accounts for 77 — 81% of the total energy expenditure. It should be recognised, therefore, that the energy cost of sedentary activities like lying and sitting is the main determinant of total energy expenditure in all but the most active people, and it is also the respect in which people differ most.

Individual variation in metabolic rate

The example of N.B. and E.T. (see page 50) shows that two individuals of the same age, sex, weight and body composition can have very different metabolic rates. The early workers on metabolic rate were mainly interested in diagnosing thyroid disease, so they tried to achieve standard 'basal' conditions, and compared the observed metabolic rate with standards based on the age, sex and surface area (calculated from the weight and height) of the subject. With modern methods for measuring body composition it has become evident that resting metabolic rate is closely related to lean body mass (Halliday et al 1979). In our experience the formula which best fits resting metabolic rate (R.M.R.) is: R.M.R. = $99.8 + (W \times 1.155) + (T.B.K. \times 0.0223) - (A \times 0.456)$ where R.M.R. is in $ml.0_2/$ minute, W is body weight (kg), T.B.K. is total body potassium (mmol) and A is age (years) (Doré et al 1981). Figure 3.9 shows the observed and predicted metabolic rate of 140 women and 9 men. The multiple correlation coefficient is 0.83, indicating that about 30% of the variability of metabolic rate among these 140 patients cannot be explained on the basis of weight, age or lean body mass.

The fact that it is possible to find a highly significant correlation between resting metabolic rate and a function of weight, age and lean body mass does not necessarily prove that these are causally associated. A more stringent test is to take a group of people in whom weight, age

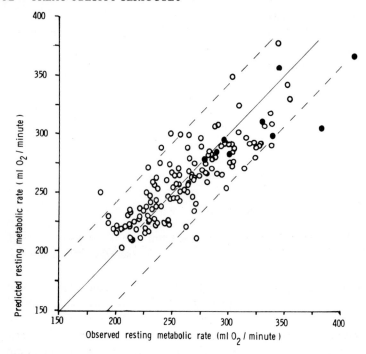

Fig. 3.9 Observed resting metabolic rate among 140 women (open circles) plotted against the metabolic rate predicted from the formula of Doré et al (1981). Closed circles show values for 9 men

and total body potassium change, and see if the change in predicted metabolic rate agrees with the observed change in metabolic rate. The result of this test in 17 women who lost 22.8 ± 13.9 kg in a year is shown in Figure 3.10. Since the average predicted change agrees so well with the average observed change, and the scatter about the line of identity is no greater than for the original equation, it becomes highly probable that weight, age and lean body mass are really factors which determine metabolic rate. Figure 3.10 also shows that the rapid decrease in metabolic rate which occurs with energy restriction (see Figure 3.2, page 22) does not continue indefinitely. After weight loss these 17 women had the metabolic rate which would have been predicted for a person of similar body composition who had not lost weight.

Diet-induced thermogenesis
One of the most hotly-disputed points concerning human obesity concerns diet-induced thermogenesis, or luxuskonsumption, to give

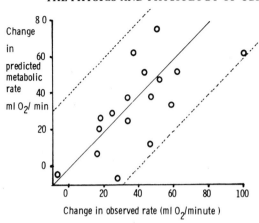

Fig. 3.10 Change in resting metabolic rate, versus change in predicted metabolic rate, among 17 women who lost 22.8 ± 13.9 kg in a year. Data of Doré et al (1981)

the old German name. Throughout the period from about 1930 to mid-1960s the idea that people burned off excess energy when overfed was regarded with great disfavour by respectable nutritionists: it was a story put about by charlatans to justify magic cures, or by self-indulgent obese people as a justification for their obesity. However the paper by Miller et al (1967) gave evidence that, in some people at least, energy expenditure increased during overeating, and thus weight gain was less than might be predicted. In the next 15 years many investigations were published which either supported or refuted the idea of dietary-induced thermogenesis. This complex literature has been reviewed elsewhere (Garrow 1978b). It is indisputable that during overfeeding the excess food cannot be accounted for by stored energy: that is clear from the work of the Vermont group (Sims et al 1973). It is not clear exactly how the excess energy expenditure is partitioned: Dauncey (1980) found an immediate increase in energy expenditure of 10% in overfed subjects, but Norgan and Durnin (1980), who also found 10% increases in metabolic rate after 42 days of overfeeding, ascribe this increase to the increase in body weight.

Recent work on overfed rats has shown that the tissue in which the increased energy expenditure takes place is brown adipose tissue (Stock 1981), and there is convincing evidence that the genetically obese strains of rodents lack the ability to raise their metabolic rate, due to a defect in their brown fat. It has also been shown that brown fat, both in animals and man, responds to infusion of noradrenalin (James 1981), and there is some evidence that obese subjects have a smaller response to noradrenalin infusions than lean subjects. Furthermore Pittet et al (1976) have shown that obese women show a smaller increase in metabolic rate after an oral load of 50 g glucose than lean women. It is possible to weave together all these observations to support the hypothesis that an important factor in obesity is the inability to produce a thermogenic response to overfeeding, so the extra energy is stored in 'metabolically obese' people as fat, but burned off in 'metabolically lean' people.

However, there are some weak links in this chain of argument. Thermoregulatory thermogenesis is much more important to a small animal, like a mouse, than it is to the large human animal, so we cannot assume that factors which are quantitatively important in rodent obesity will be quantitatively important in human obesity. The magnitude of the thermogenic response to food is always much smaller that the energy value of the food: usually about 10–15% of the meal, even in lean people. If it were true that fat and thin people had similar metabolic rates in the fasting condition, but that after a meal the lean had a higher energy expenditure than the obese, then a failure of dietary-induced thermogenesis could indeed be an important factor in obesity, but this situation does not arise. Even in the studies quoted by James (1981) the absolute energy expenditure of the obese subjects was always higher than that of the lean subjects, so failure of dietary-induced thermogenesis cannot by itself explain the obesity of these subjects.

Thermogenesis from heat, cold, exercise or anxiety

If obese people were less thermogenic, not only to food, but to a wide range of stimuli, this might make a more powerful case for the importance of this factor in the aetiology of obesity. The problem is a technically difficult one to study, since it is necessary to make a series of measurements on lean and obese subjects under strictly controlled dietary conditions. This protocol was carried out by Blaza (1980) with the results shown in Figures 3.11 and 3.12. A Latin square design was used, so each of the five lean and five obese subjects were tested in each of the experimental conditions: warm, cool, exercise, food and control. Measurement of resting metabolic rate before any of these stimuli showed that the lean subjects had a consistantly lower oxygen uptake than the obese subjects. (Figure 3.11). When lean and obese subjects performed the equivalent of 8 miles cycling on a bicycle ergometer this increased the total energy expenditure with respect to the control day, in both lean and obese subjects. An intake of an extra 800 kcal (3.4 MJ) of food caused a small increase in energy expenditure, and exposure to cool conditions increased the energy expenditure of lean subjects, but

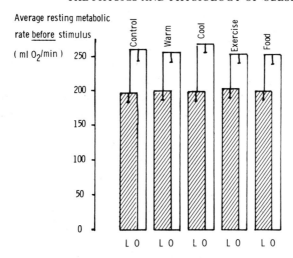

Fig. 3.11 Resting metabolic rate (Mean ± S.E.M.) among 5 lean women (shaded columns) and 5 obese women (open columns) on 5 separate days on which their response to thermogenic stimuli was tested by direct calorimetry (data of Blaza 1980)

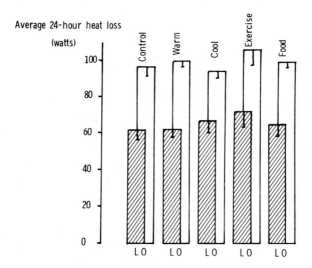

Fig. 3.12 Total 24-hour heat loss, measured by direct calorimetry, among 5 obese women (open columns) who experienced no thermogenic stimuli ('control'); the upper limit of the range of comfortable temperature ('warm'), the lower limit of comfortable temperature ('cool'), the equivalent of 8 miles cycling on a bicycle ergometer ('exercise') or and extra 800 kcal of ('food'). Data of Blaza (1980)

not of the obese ones. Under no experimental conditions did the energy expenditure of the lean subjects exceed that of the obese subjects (Figure 3.12).

These results suggest that, at least in subjects who are on a restricted energy intake, thermogenic responses to ordinary stimuli are small, and do not support the hypothesis that a failure in thermogenic responsiveness is an important factor in the aetiology of human obesity.

Attempts have also been made to measure the increase in metabolic rate caused by anxiety (Blaza and Garrow 1980). Even in circumstances which produced high resting heart rates, and significantly increased rates of excretion of catecholamines and cortisol, the increase in metabolic rate, although measurable, was small. There is no information about the relative thermogenic response to anxiety in lean and obese subjects.

HORMONES AND DRUGS AFFECTING FAT STORAGE

The energy stores of the body are in constant ebb and flow: during fasting energy is taken from these stores to supply metabolic requirements, and after feeding dietary energy goes to replenish these stores. The main site of energy storage is the fat cell: fat is formed by esterification of fatty acids and glycerol. The fatty acids from which triglyceride is formed may be synthesised within the fat cell, or may enter having been released from lipoprotein or free fatty acid which circulates bound to albumin in the plasma. The cleavage of free fatty acid from lipoprotein requires the enzyme lipoprotein lipase. The rate of entry of glucose into the fat cell, and the synthesis of fatty acid from glucose, is enhanced by the hormone insulin.

The reverse process is lipolysis: the triglyceride is split to yield fatty acid. The first step in lipolysis depends on a hormone-sensitive lipase. The activity of this enzyme is increased by catecholamines and inhibited by insulin. It is mainly the balance between the lipogenic effects of insulin and the lipolytic effects of catecholamines which regulates the flow of energy to and from the fat stores.

It may seem, from this highly simplified account, that the key to the understanding of obesity lies in these hormonal changes: given this understanding it is virtually certain that a drug could be found which would rectify the situation. However there are three important reasons for believing that it is unlikely that a breakthrough in this field will revolutionise the management of obesity.

First, it has been shown by Sims et al (1973) that the hormonal changes which are characteristic of the obese person — increased insulin concentration, decreased glucose tolerance, increased cortisol production rate, decreased growth hormone responsiveness — can all be produced in perfectly normal volunteers by experimental over-feeding. It seems, therefore, that these hormonal changes are a result, rather than a cause, of obesity.

Second, it might be that the defect in obesity was within the fat cell which, for some reason, was particularly liable to store fat. This theory has been tested in a series of experiments with various strains of genetically obese rodents (Meade et al 1979). If fat cells from genetically obese mice are transplated into lean mice the cells become smaller. If fat from the lean mice is transplanted into obese mice the transplanted cells become bigger. This is a most convincing demonstration that the metabolic abnormality of the genetically obese rodent does not reside in the fat cell itself, but in the environment of the fat cell.

Third, any explanation of obesity, or cure for obesity, must make sense in terms of energy balance. Suppose, for example, that a drug were found which increased the breakdown of fat, but had no other effect, would it be helpful in the treatment of obesity? Probably not. Suppose a person continued to eat the same amount, and expend the same amount of energy, but took this drug. Fatty acid would be mobilised from fat stores and would saturate the capacity of carrier proteins in the plasma to transport it. If still more fatty acid were now mobilised, where could it go? It must either be burned or re-esterified into fat again. It if is burned, but total energy expenditure is not increased, then the newly mobilised fatty acid will merely displace some other fuel which now will not be burned, but will be available to form new fat. There is no escape from the energy balance equation: ultimately fat stores can only be decreased if somehow energy expenditure exceeds energy intake.

However, hormones and drugs can affect energy intake and expenditure, and hence fat storage. There are well documented cases of rapid weight gain in patients who were given excessive insulin (Weiner 1980): it is important that obese diabetics are treated without insulin if possible. In the days when insulin coma was used as a treatment for depressive disease it was common to see patients becoming markedly obese. The mechanism of weight gain in this case is certainly an increased food intake.

Antidepressant and antipsychotic agents may cause weight gain: here the mechanism is not clear (Kalucy 1980). The relief of depression may remove the anorexia associated with depressive illness, and hence promote greater food intake. Alternatively the sedative effects of these drugs may decrease physical activity, and may even decrease resting metabolism. There have been no good studies on the effects of these drugs on metabolic rate.

Since catecholamines are important in stimulating lipolysis, and in some thermogenic reactions, it might be supposed that patients who were on long-term blocking agents such as propanolol would be liable to weight gain. This does not seem to be so, which is another reason for doubting the quantitative importance of thermogenesis in regulating body weight.

Oestrogens, and in particular the contraceptive pill, have been blamed for causing weight gain: this certainly happens in some women, but the mechanism is obscure. The variations in body weight and in temperature during the menstrual cycle reflect changes in body water and in the setting of thermoregulation (Bonjour et al 1978) rather than changes in metabolic rate. The most likely reason for steady weight gain in women on the contraceptive pill is increased food intake, but there is no convincing evidence on this point.

Steroids and diuretics cause transient weight change by increasing or decreasing body water respectively. There is no evidence that either class of drug affects total body fat.

The drugs most commonly administered in order to promote weight loss are thermogenic drugs, such as thyroid hormones, or anorectic drugs, which are usually related to amphetamines. The use of these agents is reviewed on pages 131–138. It should be noted that obese patients often suspect (or are told) that they have some degree of thyroid deficiency. This is rarely true. In a large series of obese and non-obese patients thyroid function tests showed a gaussian distribution in both groups, and there was no evidence that hypothyroidism was any more common among obese people than among non-obese people. (Strata et al 1978). The importance of hypothyroidism in obesity is that it reduces energy expenditure, but if metabolic rate is measured, as suggested in later chapters, this diagnosis will not be missed.

Predisposition to obesity

In the foregoing review no feature has been established which serves to differentiate obese people from lean people other than the difference in the amount of stored fat. Obese people do not systematically eat more, or absorb energy from the gut more efficiently, or expend consistantly less energy, than lean people. However the lack of a clear demarcation between fat and lean is only to be expected: if energy intake is 10% greater than energy expenditure this would lead to rapid weight gain, but there is much more than 10% variation in energy intake or expenditure among fat individuals or among lean individuals. Furthermore, it is quite possible that when we study a group of obese people only a minority have some metabolic abnormality which predisposes to obesity, and the others are obese for non-metabolic reasons. Similarly, if we studied a group of anaemic people, without any understanding of the different causes of anaemia, it is quite unlikely that deficiency of B_{12} would be detected as a cause, since such cases would be swamped by those caused by blood loss or iron deficiency.

If there is a sub-group of obese people who are particularly predisposed to obesity we might expect to find this trait among those who became obese early in life, or who had a family history of obesity. It might be that such people had a rather low metabolic rate in relation to their weight. To test this hypothesis we have plotted the resting metabolic rate against the obesity index (W/H^2) in 65 women in whom we had information about the age of onset of obesity and prevalence of obesity among their first-degree relatives (Garrow et al 1980). The results are shown in Figure 3.13. There is the expected strong correlation between W/H^2 and resting metabolic rate, but no indication that those subjects with early-onset obesity, or a family

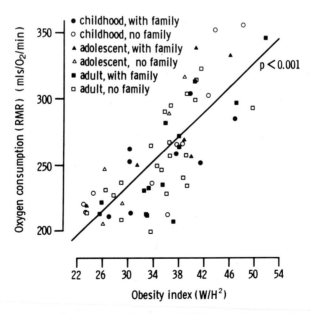

Fig. 3.13 Relation of resting metabolic rate to W/H^2 among 65 women. Symbols indicate the age of onset of obesity, and the family history of obesity. Date of Garrow et al (1980)

history of obesity, have a lower metabolic rate than their peers without these characteristics.

Björntorp and Sjöström (1979) suggest that there is a subgroup of obese people, perhaps only 0.2% of the population, who are characterised by hypercellularity of adipose tissue and who are particularly difficult to treat. On dieting they lose weight rapidly, but then rapidly regain it. It is possible that these people have some metabolic characteristic which makes it particularly difficult to maintain a reduced energy intake. Alternatively, it may be that certain obese patients are particularly 'hard cases', and that the adipose tissue hypercellularity is a consequence of their prolonged severe obesity, rather than a cause of their resistance to treatment.

Summary: energy balance in human obesity

Anyone who maintains a stable body weight over many years must somehow match energy intake and expenditure with great precision. We do not know how this is done, but there are evidently several mechanisms involved which modulate energy intake and output to achieve this balance in the long term. Short-term mechanisms are very imprecise, so most people, fat or thin, show quite wide fluctuations in energy balance. The striking difference between people who remain in the normal range, and those who become severely obese, is that the former correct errors in energy balance before they become too large, while the latter do not.

Despite intensive investigation no good evidence has been found for any defect in short-term regulation of energy balance in obese people when compared with lean people. It seems likely, therefore, that the trouble lies in the long-term regulation system, which we poorly understand. There is increasing evidence that, in man, cognitive factors are important in the regulation of body weight.

4

Investigation and treatment of grade III obesity

THE LESSER EVIL

All the methods for treating grade III obesity which are discussed in this chapter have been condemned as inhumane and senseless. It has been said that those who use such methods are motivated by a puritanical desire to punish obese people, or by cynical commercialism. These critics say that what is needed is a deeper understanding of all the physiological, psychological and social factors which lead to gross obesity, so the true cause can be tackled.

One must sympathise with these criticisms, which have some justification. It is undoubtedly true that there have been commercial exploitations of operations for the treatment of obesity, some of which have caused much litigation in the United States. In the discussion which follows some readers will no doubt remain unconvinced that such lines of treatment are ever justified: if they wish to condemn they should be specific about the alternative which they would prefer. At least the writer is in the fortunate position of being able to view the problem from a position sheltered from commercial pressures.

PREVALENCE AND NATURAL HISTORY OF GRADE III OBESITY

By definition a person with grade III obesity has a W/H^2 index over 40, so this represents a weight at least 45 kg (about 100 lb) above the maximum of the 'desirable' range of weight for height. As a rule-of-thumb we can take the energy equivalent of excess weight to be about 7000 kcal (29 MJ) per kg, so the problem is to lose at least 300,000 kcal (1300 MJ). Even with the most rapid weight loss in the range shown in Figure 2.1 (p. 12) this will take at least 10 months.

Fortunately grade III obesity is not very common. Figure 4.1 shows that a W/H^2 of 35 is the highest which is found at all frequently among employed men and women: in the survey of 2114 men and 841 women in the Northwick Park Heart Study there were none above $W/H^2 = 40$.

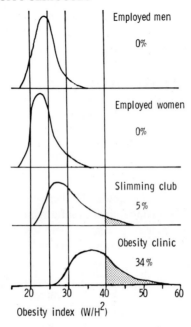

Fig. 4.1 Grade III obesity in sections of the population

However members of slimming clubs, and patients attending hospital obesity clinics show a different distribution. About 5% of the members of the Harrow Slimming Club (Seddon et al 1981), and 34% of the patients referred to the obesity clinic at Northwick Park Hospital, come in the grade III category. It is impossible to interpret these data to yield estimates of prevalence in the community, since referrals to hospital clinics are biassed by many unknown factors.

The prevalence of severe obesity in adults in the United States has been studied by Abraham and Johnson (1980), using data from the Health and Nutrition Examination Survey (HANES) on a nationwide probability sample of 28,043 persons. They define 'severe obesity' by weight or skinfold thickness, using the 95th centile values obtained on adults aged 20–29 years as the threshold for the diagnosis. The average 'severely obese' man was about 50 lb (23 kg) above average weight, and 'severely obese' women were 67 lb (30 kg) above average weight, and it was estimated that 2.8 million men and 4.5 million women in the U.S. fulfilled these criteria. However only a small proportion of these people would be sufficiently overweight to be classified as grade III obese. If we guessed that about 0.05% of the adult population was in this category it would mean about 60,000 men and women in the U.S., or about 100 people in the catchment area of a typical District General Hospital in the U.K. A general practitioner with a list of 2500 patients would probably have one such case.

Because few cases of grade III obesity will be found in random surveys of the population, our knowledge of the natural history of this condition is limited, and comes mostly from mortality statistics and experience with cases treated in hospital. Such severely obese people generally do not live very long, and the diseases to which they are particularly prone have been reviewed on page 000. It is very rare to meet a case of grade III obesity who has not been trying actively to reduce weight over the previous few years, although obviously these efforts have been unsuccessful. Usually they have been obese since childhood, but they may indicate some particular life event — marriage, pregnancy, divorce, bereavement — as a landmark at which weight gain became more rapid. However on close investigation these events prove to be punctuations in a fairly steady process of weight gain. For example a woman may say that she gained 15 kg within a few months of marriage, but then admit that she had reduced in weight by a similar amount for that occasion.

INVESTIGATION OF GRADE III OBESE PATIENTS

Severely obese patients are often pathetically willing to be investigated: they are desperate, they regard hospital referral as their last chance of successful treatment, often they have low self-esteem and consider that they must go along with whatever is suggested. This excessively docile attitude is a temptation to research workers to carry out tests far beyond the needs of diagnosis or management.

From the patients' viewpoint the facts which need to be established are as follows:

1. What is the body composition of the patient? It is known that body weight exceeds the normal range by some 45 kg (100 lb) at least, but is this excess mainly fat, or is there a large amount of excess water also?

2. What is the patient's metabolic rate? This is of importance for several reasons. First, the metabolic rate is the main determinant of total energy expenditure, especially in very obese patients who are relatively inactive (see Page 50). Second, the metabolic rate should check with predictions based on body composition: if it does not it raises the possibility of some disorder of energy metabolism. Finally, it is necessary to try to calculate the energy expenditure which the patient will have after weight reduction, because this is the factor which will be

most important in determining how easy it is to maintain the reduced weight.

3. Does the patient have any other major disability other than obesity?

If the ability of the patient to live an active independent life is anyway limited by old age, irreversible damage to weightbearing joints, chronic bronchitis, mental subnormality, or any such disability which will still exist after weight loss, then the benefit to the patient of weight loss is correspondingly reduced. In this connection the significance of depression in severely obese patients is difficult to assess: are they obese because they are depressed, or vice versa? In my experience, if there is good evidence that the patient was not very obese at the time when treatment for depression was started, it is very likely that the patient will still be depressed after weight loss. However a measure of unhappiness is a natural feature of any person disabled by obesity, and is not a contraindication to treatment. I have often been wrong in guessing to what extent depression would be improved by weight loss.

The tests which should be applied to answer questions 1 and 2 above have been described in Chapter 3. The minimum and most convenient measurements are total body potassium to assess lean body mass, and measurement of resting metabolic rate on at least three occasions as an inpatient on a reducing diet. It is useless to make random measurements of metabolic rate on outpatients on an unknown diet.

Let us suppose that the patient is a woman of 32 years, weight 115 kg, height 1.6 m, total body potassium 3000 mmol, and resting metabolic rate 300 ml O_2/minute. Her predicted metabolic rate is 285 ml O_2/minute (see Page 51) which checks well with the observed value. Her W/H^2 is 44.9, and to achieve W/H^2 of 25 she would need to weigh 64 kg, a loss of 51 kg. Her total body potassium indicates a lean body mass of 50 kg, which is quite high for a woman of her age and height, and it also implies that she has a body fat of 65 kg. At rest she will use about 2100 kcal (8.8 MJ) per day. The rule-of-thumb estimate of the energy value of her excess weight (51 kg $\times$ 7000 kcal) is that somehow she needs to expend 357,000 kcal (1500 MJ) more than she eats. This is roughly equivalent to suggesting that she should take a diet supplying 1000 kcal (4.2 MJ) per day for one year, making an allowance for the fact that her metabolic rate will decrease with weight loss.

In this example the arithmetic is favourable: there is at least a chance that by the age of 33 this woman could achieve a normal weight, with a greatly improved quality of life ahead of her. If we had chosen a woman of the same weight and height, but aged 55, with a total body potassium of 2200 mmol, and with an oxygen uptake of 210 ml/minute the outlook would be much less favourable. Her lean body mass is about 37 kg, so she is much more obese: her body fat is about 78 kg. Her daily resting energy expenditure is only about 1500 kcal (6.1 MJ) per day, so to generate an energy deficit of 357,000 kcal 1500 MJ) on a diet supplying 1000 kcal per day would take more than twice as long as for the former example. Here the arithmetic is unfavourable: she is being asked to make a much greater effort in the hope of attaining normal weight at age 57, and even at that weight she would still be more obese, and have a much lower energy requirement than the younger woman.

It is the function of a doctor to try to make life more tolerable for the patient. The jeremiads about the impossibility of treating obesity do not distinguish between those situations in which there is a good chance of obtaining worthwhile benefit (as in the first example above), and those in which quite modest objectives are appropriate (as in the second example). The actual disability suffered by the patient is relevant to the assessment of the case. If, in the second example, the woman was disabled by osteoarthritic knees, weight loss of about 15 kg would be a very sensible objective, which would be attainable, and which would bring considerable relief to the patient. In the first example (unless there was some other pathology complicating the prognosis) it would be wise to aim for a weight loss of 40 – 50 kg whether or not she had disability attributable to her obesity. Her chance of losing weight will never be greater than it is now, and if she does not lose weight the chances of developing complications will steadily increase, so there is every reason to tackle the problem vigorously as soon as possible.

Those readers who are accustomed to the American idea of a 'work-up' of the obese patient may be surprised that this section does not list tests of insulin, cortisol and catecholamine secretion, X-rays of the pituitary fossa, and so on. It is rather rarely that these tests yield abnormal results which actually help with management. Of course grossly obese people have raised plasma insulin levels, and impaired glucose tolerance: if these changes are found (or even if they are not found) I cannot see how that helps in the management of an individual patient. The more often these tests are advised in textbooks the more difficult it is for the doctor to defend himself in court against a charge of negligence if he has not done them. It is ironical that, despite batteries of tests in the 'work-up', the two that really matter — a measure of metabolic rate and of body composition — are the ones most frequently omitted.

PSYCHOLOGICAL ASSESSMENT AND SELECTION

The physical investigation of grade III patients is relatively simple and objective. Assuming that metabolically it is possible and desirable to help a given patient to lose, say, 50 kg in the course of a year, the next step is to decide if there are any insuperable psychological barriers to this course of action.

Most publications on the surgical treatment of severe obesity list as reasons for excluding patients from treatment that they are 'mentally unstable' or 'not motivated' (Yates 1980). If the patient is psychotic then any treatment for obesity will be difficult to carry out, and the results will be unsatisfactory. However the term 'mentally unstable' or 'not motivated' is capable of very wide interpretation: it could be argued that any metabolically normal person who becomes grossly obese cannot be motivated to be thin, and hence none is suitable for treatment. Innumerable attempts have been made, by administering questionnaires to outpatients, to assess motivation and predict weight loss, but none has succeeded (Rodin et al, 1977). This is not surprising, because motivation depends on expectations of benefit, and the extent to which these expectations are fulfilled.

A system for assessing grade II patients for outpatient dietary treatment is given on pages 124–128. The same principles apply in grade III, but the important difference is that, while grade II patients can afford to spend some time trying out various diets, grade III patients need to lose weight urgently before the situation deteriorates further. My own practice, therefore, is to carry out the assessment outlined on page 124 on any new grade III outpatients, and to tell the patient how much weight I think they should be able to lose, and at what rate, based on the range shown in Figure 2.1 (p. 12). If the patient rejects this as unacceptable I try to make the point that it is the best available option. If the patient says that the rate of weight loss is acceptable, but that his or her experience indicates that it will not be attained, we agree to give it another try, and see who is right when the patient returns four weeks later.

Obviously the diet which the patient takes between that first interview and the return four weeks later is crucial. If the patient 'diets' — some days more conscientiously than others — and returns having lost little weight, we have made little progress. In this situation I have found it very useful to suggest that the patient should keep to a 'milk diet' (see pages 68 and 95). The return visit is then bound to be informative. The possibilities are as follows:

1. The patient comes back having lost between 4 and 8 kg, encouraged by this progress, and saying that it was not as difficult as

expected to keep to milk. So long as this happy state of affairs continues it is merely necessary to see the patient monthly and provide guidance and encouragement.

2. The patient comes back having lost only about 2 kg, and saying that he or she found the diet impossibly boring after a few days. In principle the idea of the milk diet is acceptable, but in practice the temptation to eat is too strong. It is then necessary to see if this temptation can be reduced. Is the patient a housewife who continues to cook for her family? Does she work in a catering establishment? Do her family taunt her about her inability to diet, and do they realise that it will be to their disadvantage if she cannot do the housework? Whatever the problem, can the situation be improved so it is worth having another try? It is worth trying to alter the domestic situation, since this is the environment to which the patient will return, even if it is decided that jaw-wiring is a desirable option. The easier it is made for the patient to diet at home the greater are the chances of a successful outcome in the end.

If it appears that there is no hope of getting the patient to keep to milk at home, and if he or she is set on some form of surgical intervention, it is best to admit the patient to a metabolic ward for assessment.

3. The patient returns having lost only about 2 kg, but insisting that the milk diet has been strictly adhered to. In this situation the patient should be admitted, because if the story is true it indicates an unusual metabolism. If, on admission, it proves to be untrue this saves subsequent misunderstandings.

4. The patient does not return. In this situation it is likely that the patient was unimpressed by the treatment offered, and is opting either for different treatment elsewhere, or for no treatment. It is my practice to write to the referring doctor explaining the situation, and expressing willingness to see the patient should his or her assessment of priorities change. Quite frequently such patients make a new appointment a year or so later, having discovered for themselves, often at considerable expense, that magic cures do not work.

STAGES OF TREATMENT FOR GRADE III OBESITY

An important principle in medicine is *primum non nocere*. Therefore those lines of treatment should first be considered which are least likely to harm the patient. On these grounds the milk diet must come top of the list.

A milk diet

Three imperial pints (1800 ml) of ordinary whole cow's milk provides 1170 kcal (4.9 MJ) and 59 g of protein of high biological quality. It is cheap and readily available almost anywhere. It is deficient in iron, vitamins and fibre, but these deficiencies can easily be made up by one multivitamin capsule BPC and 200 mg ferrous sulphate daily, and an inert bulk laxative if necessary.

For the severely obese person, who has failed many times with diets, milk has several advantages. The reasons which patients give for failing to keep to diets are numerous:

1. 'It was too much trouble to prepare special salads.' No one can say that milk is trouble to prepare.

2. 'The diet was too expensive.' It would be hard to find a diet cheaper than milk.

3. 'I could not be bothered to weigh out portions.' No weighing is necessary with milk: either two or three pints is the ration, and when it is finished it is finished.

4 'I could not get the diet foods when I went out.' If the patients are not sufficiently serious about dieting to go out only to places where it is acceptable to drink milk, then they are not serious enough.

5 'The diet was too monotonous.' Milk is indeed very monotonous, but it is unlikely that the patient will find any diet which is gastronomically satisfying and also produces the necessary weight loss.

6 'I would cheat myself on the diet, pretending that extra items today would be compensated by eating less tomorrow, but that never happened.' With the milk diet the rules are so simple that self-deception of this sort is easily avoided.

The milk diet does not, of course, solve all the problems of treating grade III obesity, but it clarifies them. Some patients, particularly older ones, lose perhaps 10–15 kg in about 4–6 months, obtain symptomatic relief from painful joints and shortness of breath, and settle for that. The more difficult problem is the young patient in whom the objective is to achieve 40–50 kg weight loss, because this involves keeping to the milk diet for 10 months or more. Relatively few patients achieve this. When they are about to give up the continuation of treatment depends on the reasons for giving up, and how near to the target weight they have come.

It is an advantage to run a clinic at which some patients have their jaws wired, because other patients can talk to them and get first-hand advice about the advantages and disadvantages of this line of treatment. Most patients who have their jaws wired find it far less stressful than relying on their own determination to keep to milk only, and thus other patients tend to opt for this line of treatment.

Jaw wiring

It is well known that whenever a new method of treatment is introduced, medical colleagues immediately do two things — first they modify the treatment, then they publish articles saying it does not work. Kopp (1975) provides a good example of this approach. He reports the case of a woman who weighed 127 kg (280 lb) who asked to have her jaws fixed to help her to diet. He did this with arch-bars fitted to the posterior teeth, but insisted on removing these fortnightly to clean the teeth. She lost 20 kg (43 lb) in 4 months, but then they decided to remove the fixation for two weeks. Shortly after it was replaced following this respite, she said she could not tolerate it and had it removed. Kopp therefore concludes that this mode of treatment is useless.

I started treating obese patients by jaw wiring in 1973 because I was impressed by how hard it is for outpatients to keep to a reducing diet, especially when they have already achieved substantial weight loss, but how relatively easy the same patients find it to keep to a diet when confined to a metabolic ward. It is exhausting and frustrating every day to be confronted with the responsibility of deciding not to eat food which any normal person can eat freely. If the responsibility is taken away, because the food is not accessible, it is a relief. Prolonged inpatient treatment for obesity is impossibly expensive in hospital resources, and it is disruptive to the life of the patient to be removed from society for many months. Ideally the patients might reorganise their own homes and places of work so that it presented no dietary temptations, but this is seldom practicable.

The rationale behind jaw wiring, therefore, is to try to interpose a barrier which will protect the patient from directly accessible food. Jaw wiring will not in itself guarantee adherence to a diet — anything the patient might have wished to eat can easily be homogenised and taken through wired jaws — but it does mean that the patient has to take some deliberate action to frustrate the purpose of the wires, such as homogenising food or removing the wires. However, to help the patient to feel that the wires are a secure protection against the impulse to binge, it seems obvious that the wires should be disturbed as little as possible. In our experience (Fordyce et al 1979), provided the condition of teeth and gums is good when fixation is applied, only milk is drunk, and the mouth is kept clean by the regular use of mouthwashes, no deterioration in dental condition occurs during periods of fixation up to 12 months. Wood (1977) was concerned about the stiffening of the tempormandibular joint and periodontal disease during long periods of jaw fixation. He therefore used metal cap splints on the teeth, which were unlocked every few weeks to inspect the teeth, measure the maximum opening of the mouth, and to prevent the patients developing 'a dependance on the splints for regulation of the diet': Wood thinks obese patients have a 'gluttinous nature and temperament', and has evidently fallen into the trap of thinking that all one has to do with grade III obese patients is to teach them to eat 'normally'. Of course this is not so: to generate an energy deficit which is reflected in a weight loss of 24 kg in 6 months (the result he reports) requires a food intake about 1000 kcal (4.2 MJ) less than 'normal' —i.e. the intake which would just match requirements. It is surprising that his patients tolerated this regimen. The study had the merit of showing that there was no detrimental change in dental tissues during this period of fixation. If fixation is applied continuously for 9–12 months the patients are usually unable to open the mouth fully immediately after the wires are removed, but full mobility of the jaws is regained within one week in our experience. In view of the psychological trauma involved in removal and replacement of the fixation it causes less trouble to leave the wires in place.

The report of Drenick and Hargis (1978) draws attention to the danger of aspiration of vomit in a person with wired jaws: their patients were provided with wire cutters and instructed to cut the wires in an emergency. We have preferred a policy of fixing the teeth with enough space to permit clearance of the airway in such a situation. It is of little practical help to expect patients, or their relatives, to unwire a patient who is vomiting, since this is quite a difficult thing to do quickly, and to suggest that it might be necessary must undermine the confidence of the patient.

Selection of patients for jaw wiring is on the basis that they have tried a diet of milk for some weeks or months, cannot keep to this any longer, but still need and want to lose weight. However there is little benefit to the patient in weight loss if this weight is rapidly gained when the wires are removed. When I started jaw wiring I believed patients who thought that they had learned to control the impulse to overeat. I now know that this optimism is usually unjustified: most will regain weight unless something is done to stop it (Fordyce et al 1979, Drenick and Hargis 1978). Therefore the decision to opt for jaw wiring is a package deal in which the patient agrees to three conditions:

1 The fixation will remain in place until there is no medical indication for further weight loss.

2 The patient will attend monthly for outpatient supervision.

3 When the wires are removed a nylon cord will be fixed round the waist of the patient so it is comfortable if weight loss is maintained, but not if weight is regained.

Thus the patient is discouraged from 'trying out' jaw wiring: if he or she decides that the assistance of jaw wiring is required this decision must be regarded as irrevocable, not tentative.

This arrangement may be critisised on the grounds that it is too paternalistic, but in effect the agreement is very similar to that which a patient makes when consenting to a bypass operation. If a patient consents to jaw wiring, but would refuse a bypass operation, because the operation carries a higher risk, this is a sensible judgement. However if jaw wiring is preferred because it more easily leaves the patient with the option of changing his or her mind this is a different matter. So long as the patient has lingering doubts that weight loss could be achieved without any surgical procedure that patient should be encouraged to continue to use 'willpower'.

The package deal also puts great responsibilities on the doctor. It is essential that the investigations outlined in section 4.c are carried out, otherwise a situation may occur in which the patient is losing weight very slowly, and the expected benefits from jaw wiring are not being delivered. Provided patients are selected who have a genuine medical need to lose weight, a reasonable body composition, and a fairly high resting metabolic rate this embarrassing situation need not arise. In the case of patients with a resting oxygen consumption less than 240 ml/minute the decision to proceed to jaw wiring should be made with great caution, and the patient should be warned that weight loss will not be rapid. If the oxygen uptake is less than 200 ml/minute it is doubtful if it is ever wise to attempt jaw wiring. I have never done so, and cannot think of circumstances in which it would be the best available option.

The technique of jaw wiring is illustrated in Figure 4.2. After careful examination of the teeth, and treatment of any caries or gum infection, eyelets of thin stainless steel wire are prepared as shown at (a), and passed between the molar teeth (b). The ends of the wires encircle two adjacent teeth and are secured by being twisted together (c). Eyelets are fixed close to the gum margin, usually two pairs on each side of the mouth. Stainless steel wire of a heavier guage is laced through pairs of eyelets (d) and secured (e).

The short-term complication from this procedure is pain which may originate in four ways. First, the gums may be bruised, or one of the circumferential wires may be pressing on the edge of the gum, rendering it ischaemic. Second, the teeth may ache as a result of the sideways force on them. Third, there may be a spasm of the masseter muscle which occurs reflexly when the jaw cannot be opened normally. These three sources of discomfort can all be avoided if the patient is given a sedative dose of diazepam (usually 20 mg, repeated twice if necessary) orally immediately after the wires have been applied. This

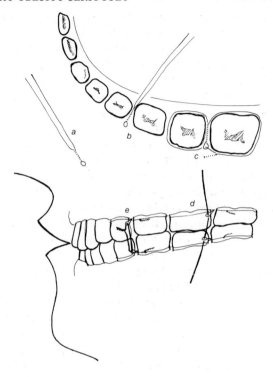

Fig. 4.2 Technique of jaw wiring. For explanation see text

prevents muscle spasm, and enables the patient to sleep until the pain from teeth and gums has subsided, which usually takes about 12–24 hours. A fourth source of discomfort may occur two to four days after wiring: this is ulceration of the buccal surface of the lip by a protruding loop of wire. However carefully the wires are applied there may be slight movement in the first two days which causes an end of wire to protrude. The patient should be warned to report immediately local tenderness from this cause, which can be treated by pushing the wire out of the way, and perhaps smoothing the surface with dental wax while the mucosa recovers. There are no long-term complications other than those associated with massive weight loss for any reason (Rodgers et al 1977, Harding 1980). If it is necessary for the management of respiratory tract infections to release the fixation this can be done by removing the vertical tie wires, but without interfering with the eyelets.

Alternative methods of fixation may be used for patients with poor dentition (Goss 1979). By means of metal cap splints it is possible to achieve satisfactory fixation in almost any patient, but this system involves more dental work, and is aesthetically less satisfactory if it is necessary to cover the incisor teeth with cap splints.

Dubois and Fizer (1978) have reported psychosexual dysfunction in patients with fixed jaws, but we have not had this experience, perhaps because the patients were so carefully informed and prepared for the implications of the procedure. It is essential that the spouse of the patient should also be informed and agree to the procedure.

Most published series report wire breakages, and there is always doubt if this is accidental or deliberate. It is important that the dentist should use much heavier wire to fix the jaws of obese patients than is used for fixing fractured jaws (Fordyce et al 1979). The patient with a fractured jaw is inhibited by pain from using much force to move the jaws, but in the obese patient the normal muscles can exert very severe pressures during yawning or sneezing. Breakage of wires is unsettling both for the patient and dentist, and it is better to overestimate than to underestimate the gauge of wire to use.

The main criticism of jaw wiring has been that after unwiring weight is regained (Drenick and Hargis 1978, Harding 1980). It is to guard against this that the waist cord is fitted. At the time of unwiring patients are very confident that they will not regain weight, because they have had the experience of relatively effortless weight loss over the previous months. If some weight gain occurs it tends to pass unnoticed: they are still far thinner than before, and have plenty of clothes which fit easily. Thus patients will return to outpatient clinics with a gain of a few kilogrammes which is regarded as a temporary phase: they tend to put off the day when a real effort is made to lose weight until many kilogrammes have been gained, and at that stage the task is too difficult. With the waist cord attention is focussed on weight gain of more than about 6 kg — it cannot be ignored, so the patient is forced to decide either to lose the extra weight or to cut the cord. Few will take the latter course, since it is an act deliberately frustrating an objective which they desire, namely to attain and maintain a normal weight. Figure 4.3 illustrates the weight curve of patients during and after jaw wiring, with and without a waist cord (Garrow and Gardiner 1981).

Gastric reduction

The history of the development of this operation is well described by Mason et al (1980). The original operation devised by Mason and Ito (1967) was patterned on the Billroth II gastrectomy (Figure 4.4 A). The stomach is transected, and a gastroenterostomy is made with a small stoma (a, Figure 4.4) between the fundus of the stomach and a loop of jejunum. This is a difficult operation to perform in a massively

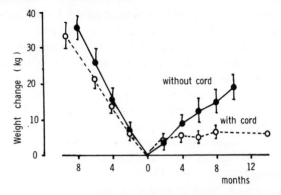

Fig. 4.3 Weight change (Mean ± S.E.M.) during and after jaw wiring, showing the effect of a waist cord on the maintenance of weight loss (Data of Garrow and Gardiner 1981)

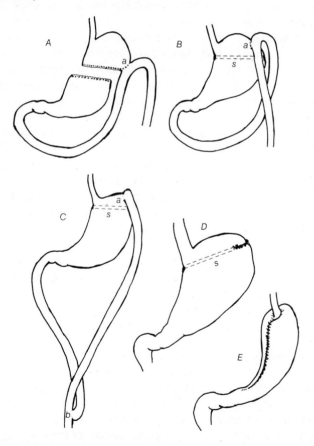

Fig. 4.4 Various versions of gastric reduction operations. For explanation see text

obese patient, since the anastamosis has to be made high in the dome of the diaphragm, which is an inaccessible region in such patients. Furthermore, experience showed that in many patients the operation did not reduce food intake severely enough, or for long enough, to obtain the desired weight loss.

The advent of stapleing techniques made the operation much easier, so the operation shown at B, Figure 4.4, became favoured. The stomach is not transected, and thus there is not the same anxiety about leakage from anastomoses. Instead a line of staples (s) is used to close off the lower part of the stomach, and the anastamosis is made as before at (a).

A disadvantage of the operation shown at B, Figure 4.4, is that bile from the jejunum is liable to reflux into the stomach and predispose to oesophagitis, so the Roux-en-Y modification was developed, shown at Figure 4.4 C. This involves an additional anastomosis at (b).

A simpler version of the operation was proposed by Gomez (1980), illustrated at Figure 4.4 D. Here the stomach is partitioned by a row of staples (s) to form a very small pouch, with a capacity of only 60 ml, which communicates through a stoma formed round a 12 mm bougie, and reinforced with a ring suture of non-absorbable material so it cannot distend. Finally, Figure 4.4 E shows yet another technique for reducing the capacity of the stomach by folding it upon itself and preventing it from enlarging by wrapping it in plastic mesh (Wilkinson 1980).

The objective of all these operations is similar to that of jaw wiring — to prevent the patient from taking large meals. In the case of gastric reduction procedures, once the small gastric pouch is full further food intake must be accommodated in the oesophagus, and when that is full the patient will choke. It is claimed that the operation enhances satiety (Villar et al 1979).

The disadvantage of the gastric reduction operation as a means of treating severe obesity is that the surgical procedure (itself a hazard for very obese patients) is being asked to do two jobs: first to reduce food intake below requirements so as to achieve weight loss, and second, to limit intake after weight loss so a normal weight will be maintained. There is no doubt that the more severe versions, with a small gastric pouch and a very small stoma through which the food has to pass, will do the first job. If it will achieve the second, time alone will tell. It is obvious that no surgical procedure can guarantee maintenance at normal weight. Let us suppose that the patient needs 2000 kcal (8.4 MJ) daily to maintain weight: whatever size the stoma or the fundal pouch it would always be possible to take a little more, or a little less, than requirements. If it was 5% more, then over the years those extra 100 kcal (420 kJ) would accumulate as gained fat. The only device which monitors small cumulative positive errors in energy balance is the bathroom scales, or indeed, the waist cord.

An alternative strategy is to use the gastric bypass as a follow-up procedure to jaw wiring in those patients for whom the waist cord is an unacceptable method for monitoring weight gain. It is now being asked to do only one job: to assist in preventing weight gain, and the operation is technically easier and safer on patients who are no longer grossly obese (Fordyce et al 1979).

ALTERNATIVE TREATMENTS FOR GRADE III OBESITY

The sequence: milk diet — jaw wiring with waist cord — gastric bypass, seems to offer the best programme for the severely obese patient. However only a minority of patients are treated in this way, so it is necessary to review alternative lines of treatment.

Jejunoileal bypass

This operation was conceived with the benign intention of enabling the obese patient to eat as much as he liked, but still to cause him to lose weight, since the food would not be digested or absorbed. This seems to be exactly what the patient wants, so the operation has been very popular. The stages in the evolution of the operation are shown in Figure 4.5. The original operation, in which the first 35 cm of jejunum is anastomosed end-to-side with the last 10 cm of ileum, is shown at Figure 4.5 A. There was a tendency for food to reflux up the blind loop of ileum, so the operation was changed to an end-to-end anastomosis, with the bypassed ileum being drained into the colon (B). This did not solve the problem of the growth of abnormal flora in the large blind loop, so a further modification is to join the proximal end of the blind loop to the gall bladder (C) so it is no longer a blind loop, or even to make two parallel alimentary tracts (D) one from the stomach to the caecum and the other from the proximal duodenum to the caecum (Hallberg 1980, Scopinaro et al 1980). These later modifications increase the technical difficulty of the operation, and leave more cut ends of bowel which are potential sites of trouble postoperatively.

The short-term mortality and morbidity of the jejunoileal bypass operation depends greatly on the skill and experience of those undertaking the procedure. It is unfortunate that the original operation (Figure 4.5 A) is technically fairly easy, and hence was attempted by many surgeons with little experience in coping with the severe metabolic problems which follow the operation. During the passage through 45 cm (18 inches) of small bowel digestion and

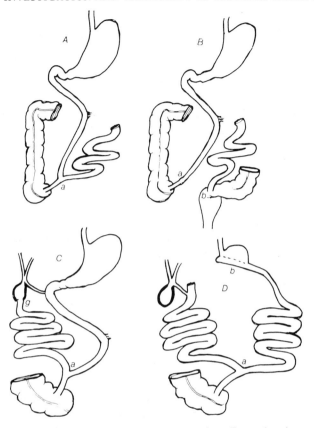

Fig. 4.5 Various versions of jejunoileal bypass operations. For explanation see text

absorption of fat is minimal: this is the primary objective of the operation. However if fat is split as far as fatty acid, and free fatty acid enters the large bowel, this in turn affects the absorption from the bowel of fat-soluble vitamins, calcium, magnesium, oxalate and water. If fat is not absorbed, fat-soluble vitamins are not absorbed either. If free fatty acids are not absorbed they form insoluble soaps with calcium and magnesium, which is therefore not absorbed. The oxalate, which would normally be bound to calcium and therefore not absorbed, is now free, and is absorbed. Finally, since a high osmotic load is presented to the large bowel this causes diarrhoea, which the patient learns to control by reducing fluid intake. This enhances the chance that oxalate stones will form in the kidney, since more oxalate than normal is being absorbed, and there is less water to keep it in solution in the urine, since less is being taken in and more is being lost in the faeces.

It should be noted that many of these problems arise because food is mixed with bile and pancreatic enzymes, and then almost immediately dumped into the large bowel, which is not adapted to cope with this mixture. The reasoning behind the bilio-pancreatic bypass (Scopinaro et al 1980), shown in Figure 4.5 D, is to avoid these problems by providing one passage for food, without pancreatic admixture, and another for bile and pancreatic secretion, the two to join only just before, or even at, the caecum. The bile salts are absorbed before they meet the food, so the unabsorbed fat enters the large bowel as neutral fat, not fatty acid. This alleviates the problems relating to water and electrolyte absorption, but it seems that two complications are inevitable in any operation designed to impair the digestion and absorption of food. First, if the fat is not digested and absorbed it will never be possible to have normal absorption of the fat-soluble vitamins. Second, and probably more important, if most of the energy-containing elements in the diet are presented to the large bowel these will sustain a greatly increased fermentation by large-bowel bacteria. It is a mistake to believe that any significant part of the diet, even the so-called 'unavailable carbohydrate', is excreted unchanged in the faeces. Most of the solid matter in faeces is bacterial, and these bacteria obtain the energy necessary for growth by fermentation of unabsorbed material from the diet. This fermentation produces gas, notably hydrogen and methane.

Fortunately, weight loss in patients with jejunoileal bypass is not attributable in any major degree to malabsorption of the diet, but to reduced food intake. It has been convincingly shown (Pilkington et al 1976, Bray et al 1976a) that after the bypass operation patients reduce food intake considerably. The reason for this change in eating habits is not clear (Robinson et al 1979, Rodin 1980). The operation radically alters the sequence of events which normally trigger the release of gut hormones after a meal, but it is impossible to say to what extent such physiological signals, or alterations in taste or perception of food, or mere learned avoidance of eating behaviour which leads to diarrhoea, contribute to the observed reduction in food intake.

Vagotomy without drainage
If the vagus nerve is cut gastric secretion and motility is reduced. This effect has been used by Kral (1980) to treat severely obese patients. He reports a mean weight loss of 19.6 kg in 7 patients after follow-up from 6–18 months. The patients report absence of hunger, and eat for purely social reasons. The effect of vagotomy in slowing gastric emptying, and reducing food intake, has been well documented in experimental animals. On theoretical grounds it may prove to be a

valuable method for treating severe obesity, but longer follow-up is required to see if there are unforeseen complications.

Inpatient starvation

The procedure which causes the greatest energy deficit, and the most rapid weight loss, is total starvation. However prolonged starvation has been associated with several cases of sudden death, probably as a result of excessive loss of lean tissue. Therefore inpatient supervision is essential, and this involves a large investment of time, money, and medical manpower (Drenick 1976). The long-term results do not justify this investment. Proximal myopathy in starving patients has recently been reported (Scorbie et al 1980). After starvation weight is usually rapidly regained (Maagøe and Mogensen 1970). Total starvation is now used mainly by commercial weight-reduction organisations who need impressive short-term results to justify the fees charged. It is hard to find any justification for this line of treatment from the viewpoint of the patient.

Inpatient semi-starvation on a diet which meets the criteria set out on page 90 is very satisfactory as a method for reducing the fat content of obese patients: indeed the most impressive feats of weight loss have been achieved by this method (Bortz 1969). The disadvantage is the great cost in providing inpatient treatment for long enough to achieve a worthwhile weight loss. Patients who want to come into hospital 'to start me off on a reducing diet' imagine that a period of a few weeks supervised dieting may make it easier to continue on the diet at home. There is no evidence that this is so: probably the contrary is true. In a well-run ward the patient will lose, say, 5 kg in 3 weeks, and will leave thinking that dieting is easy. At home it will be evident that dieting is not easy, and even if the diet is observed strictly the rate of weight loss does not match that attained in the first few weeks, for reasons set out on page 20. Thus inpatient treatment of a patient who has never seriously tried to diet is counterproductive. Sometimes, for a patient who has been dieting, but who has now ceased to lose weight, it is useful to demonstrate by inpatient treatment that weight loss is still possible. In any case the most difficult problem concerns the maintenance of weight loss, which is discussed in the next section.

Panniculectomy

It is not strictly true to say that the only way in which an obese patient can lose fat is to have a smaller energy intake than energy output, and hence burn fat to make up the deficit in energy balance. An alternative plan is to have the fat excised. This may seem an attractive proposition to someone who is very conscious of about 20 kg of excess adipose tissue hanging like an apron from the abdominal wall — to lose all this fat without even having to diet seems very desirable.

Unfortunately the results of panniculectomy are very disappointing. The pannus adiposus, or layer of subcutaneous fat, may well reach a thickness of 50 mm in an obese person who has about 50 kg of excess fat to lose. Suppose this fat layer is excised over a circle of 300 mm in diameter the volume of fat removed would be about 3.5 litres, and its weight about 3.2 kg. In order to get this fat out the area of skin undermined would be about 700 cm^2, which is very large compared with, for example, a total mastectomy. The morbidity associated with an operation of this magnitude is a high price to pay for the loss of so little fat, and the cosmetic result after the healing of the large skin flaps is seldom satisfactory.

Cosmetic reduction of excess abdominal skin after weight loss is a much more worthwhile operation. In young patients the skin of the neck, upper arms and thighs remodels very well after massive weight loss, and no surgical intervention is needed, but large flaps of abdominal skin can be neatly removed leaving an inconspicuous scar.

FOLLOW-UP AND MAINTENANCE OF WEIGHT LOSS

A comparison of the various modes of treatment for grade III obesity is set out in Table 4.1. All the treatments give good weight loss initially, but those which involve bowel bypass carry a short-term mortality from the anaesthetic and operation. The milk diet does worst so far as compliance is concerned. In the patient who has had some operation to restrict food intake compliance is virtually forced. Inpatient starvation involves uncertain compliance, depending on the strictness of supervision of the patients.

In the long term the results of the milk diet are poor because compliance is poor. We are not sure if in the long term the application of a waist cord will greatly improve the results after jaw wiring. Gastric reduction has the best proven record for long-term results, but it has not yet been followed for as long as the jejunoileal bypass procedure.

Jejunoileal bypass is coming under increasing criticism as a result of long-term complications. For example Buckwalter (1980) says

'Jejunoileal bypass is no longer an acceptable or defensible operation because of the prohibitive morbidity — liver failure, malnutrition, enteritis, oxalate urinary tract stones, arthritis and osteomalacia — and the expense related to postoperative outpatient and inpatient care, long term follow-up, and symptoms caused by the diarrhoea that seriously interfere with the quality of the patient's life'.

The newer modifications of the bypass operation may improve this

Table 4.1 Short-term and long-term results of different methods for treating grade III obesity

| Treatment | Short-term | | Long-term | | | Comments |
	Weight loss	Safety	Compliance	Weight loss	Safety	
Milk diet	Good	Good	Poor	Poor	Good	Worth trying
Jaw wiring	Good	Good	Good	?	Good	Waist cord may assist maintenance of weight loss
Gastric reduction	Good	Moderate	Good	Good	Good	Best used after jaw wiring
Jejunoileal bypass	Good	Moderate	Good	Good	Poor	Too many long-term dangers
Vagotomy	Good	Fairly good	Good	?	?	Promising: more data needed
Inpatient starvation	Good	Fairly good	?	Poor	Moderate	Expensive and ineffective in the long term

melancholy picture, but on present evidence gastric reduction is a better option.

We do not have enough long-term data to judge vagotomy against the other procedures, but so far it is promising. Long-term inpatient starvation is justified only in very special circumstances.

It is obvious from this brief review that long-term follow-up is essential in the treatment of severe obesity. Short-term weight loss is no guide to the outcome. It is unfortunate that the condition which most urgently requires careful follow-up by a competent physician is jejunoileal bypass, since several thousand patients per year have had this operation since it became popular in 1974 (Anderson et al 1980). The publicity implied that once the operation was complete the obese patient need not worry about dieting, but would achieve effortless weight loss. The reality has proved very different, since increasingly late complications are being described. 'The surgeon who performs jejunoileal bypass has the responsibility to insure adequate follow-up for his patients for the duration of their lives' (Buckwalter 1980). This is impossible unless each surgeon stops when he has done the number of cases which he personally can follow. Even if this ideal were applied it would bring further problems, because the operation would no longer be done by the surgeons who were experienced in the procedure, and less experienced surgeons would take their place.

For long-term weight loss there is little to choose between jejunoileal bypass or the various gastric reduction operations. Table 4.2 sets out the results reported in several recent series. There is more long-term information about jejunoileal bypass, because it has been used widely since 1974: there are no 5-year data on the biliopancreatic

Table 4.2   Weight loss on long-term follow-up of obese patients with various operations

Operation	n	Follow-up (years)	Weight loss (kg)	Reference
Jejunoileal bypass	1711	1	46	Andersen et al 1980
	74	1	41	Buchwald 1980
	44	1	35	Faloon et al 1980
Gastric bypass	243	1	31	Mason et al 1980
Gastroplasty	48	1	54	Gomez 1980
Bilio-pancreatic bypass	22	1	29	Scopinaro et al 1980
Vagotomy	4	1	20	Kral 1980
Bilio-pancreatic bypass	4	2	35	Scopinaro et al 1980
Jejunoileal bypass	346	5	50	Andersen et al 1980
	11	5	40	Faloon et al 1980
Gastric bypass	29	5	35	Mason et al 1980

bypass or on vagotomy. The survey by Yates (1980) of physicians supplying answers to a questionnaire about jejunoileal or gastric bypass showed that the two procedures were deemed similar in success and failure rate, and in cost: about $U.S. 6000 was the average, ranging from $3000 to $20,000, but mortality and morbidity were rather higher for jejunoileal bypass.

5

Treatment of grade II obesity

PREVALENCE AND NATURAL HISTORY OF GRADE II OBESITY

Cases of grade II obesity have, by definition, an obesity index between 30 and 40. The advantages of this arbitrary classification have been reviewed on page 3, and the uses and limitations of the obesity index (W/H^2) have been discussed on page 27: these arguments will not be repeated here.

It is not easy to obtain reliable data about the prevalence of people in this category in the general population. The distribution curves for obesity index in various subsets of the population in the Harrow Health District is shown in Figure 5.1: among 2114 employed men 4% were in the grade II range, and among 841 employed women the proportion in the range was 5%, but in both cases the numbers decrease greatly in the upper part of the range. In the survey by the American Cancer Society (Lew & Garfinkel 1979) of 336,442 men and 419,060 women the weights are reported relative to the average weight for each sex-height-age group, but from the data it is possible to calculate that about 8% of the men and 3% of the women had an index over 30. It is probably reasonable to estimate that about 4% of the population in the UK and USA have grade II obesity, so a general practitioner with 1000 adult patients would expect to have about 40 such patients: this figure agrees reasonably well with the prevalence reported by Binnie (1977). A hospital serving a population of 250,000 would expect to have 10,000 such patients in its catchment area. Cases of grade II obesity form 61% of the patients attending the Northwick Park Hospital obesity clinic and 42% of the members of the Slimming Club (Seddon et al 1981).

The data of Hartz and Rimm (1980) on members of the slimming organisation 'TOPS' expresses obesity in terms of percent above ideal weight. On the assumption that the ideal weight for women is equivalent to an obesity index $W/H^2 = 20.6$ (West 1980) it is possible to recalculate the weight groups in terms of obesity index: less than

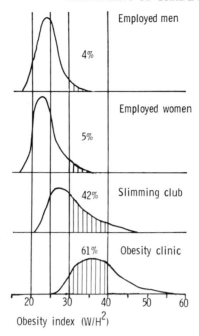

Fig. 5.1 Grade II obesity in sections of the population

20% overweight agrees fairly well with the grade 0 category, 20–50% overweight is nearly equivalent to grade I obesity, 50–100% is nearly equivalent to grade II, and over 100% is grade III. Using this conversion the proportion of members in categories 0 to III is 21%, 57%, 38% and 5% which agrees well with the distribution of the Harrow Slimming Club members who were 10%, 43%, 42% and 5% in grades 0, I, II, and III respectively (Seddon et al 1981).

The natural history of grade II obesity is difficult to describe since individuals take very different paths. In the series of Hartz and Rimm (1980) there was no common theme in the previous weight history of women who were overweight at age 50–59 years. At any previous age some had been overweight and some had not, nor is there any common landmark at which obesity is particularly likely to develop. In such a heterogeneous group it is impossible to make useful generalisations about the aetiology and development of obesity, but individual case reports are sometimes illuminating. Figure 5.2 illustrates the weight history of a middle-aged woman with grade II obesity over the course of 8 years. In 1972, at the age of 47, she began seriously to worry about her obesity. She visited various doctors, and was put on thyroxine for alleged thyroid deficiency. She then moved to a different district,

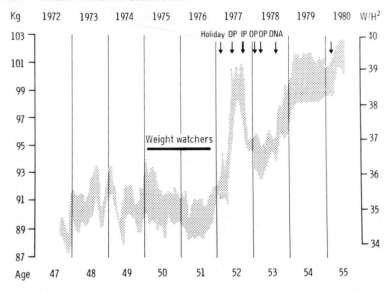

Fig. 5.2 Weight history of a case of grade II obesity. (For description see text)

where her new doctor discontinued her thyroxin, but she started to keep a record of her weight each morning, since she was impressed by the day-to-day variations. The weight record was kept in a book, and not graphically, so she was unaware of the longer-term trends which are obvious in Figure 5.2.

During 1972 to 1974 it is evident that the day-to-day variation involves swings of about 2 kg, but there are longer fluctuations, particularly involving weight gain before and during the holiday season at Christmas and during the late summer, followed by weight loss. However there is a slight upward movement, so that after Christmas 1974, which was associated with a particularly rapid weight gain, she joined the slimming organisation Weight Watchers. She kept faithfully attending until shortly before Christmas 1976, and during this period her weight fell slightly, and showed smaller seasonal fluctuations. In early 1977 family illness placed a great strain upon her, and she relaxed her diet and, as might be expected, gained some weight. However the crucial moment came when she went abroad with her daughter on holiday for 3 weeks, ate with abandon, and returned to find that she had lost 6 lb (3 kg) in weight.

At this point she became completely disenchanted with any idea of dietary restriction, since she observed that 3 weeks of self-indulgence had achieved as great a weight loss as nearly two years of conscientious weight-watching. However throwing off the shackles of diet was associated with a precipitous weight gain to about 100 kg in April 1977. Her doctor referred her to the clinic at Northwick Park Hospital, where it was agreed that if her metabolism was such that she only lost weight when eating excessively (which was the version of her history she believed at that time) this was a phenomenon worthy of investigation. She agreed to adopt a moderate diet until it was possible to admit her, and her weight was fairly stable until August 1977 when she became an inpatient.

On a standard 3.4 MJ (800 kcal) diet she lost 3 kg in 3 weeks, which is rather less than average. Her metabolic rate was rather low (190 ml/min oxygen uptake), but there was no evidence of hypothyroidism. She was considerably troubled by osteoarthritis of the knees, and her W/H^2 was about 39, so she was perilously close to the border of grade III obesity. In view of all this she agreed to try a diet of only 2 pints (1200 ml) of milk daily with the usual iron and vitamin supplements (see page 68). She went home and attended the hospital as an outpatient in January and March 1978 showing good progress with weight loss. Since she lived far from the hospital she asked for another appointment in August 1978, but did not attend. She reappeared at the hospital in March 1980 having regained all the weight she had lost, and was readmitted in June 1980 when her investigations showed the same results as before. It was at this stage that she produced the weight-record books from which Figure 5.2 has been constructed.

This case has been reviewed at some length because it is unusual for a patient with grade II obesity to keep so meticulous a weight record over such a long period. It is also instructive because it shows that the same person will undergo several changes in attitude to her weight problem. During 1972, when the record began, she was interested in the metabolic significance of relatively small changes in weight, particularly in reference to the menstrual cycle. This changed to concern about her weight and its effect on her arthritis after the rapid weight gain of Christmas 1974, and this caused her to join Weight Watchers. Had it not been for the domestic crisis in late 1976 she might have stabilised her weight at about 90 kg: even with this she might have regained control of the situation if it had not been for paradoxical weight loss during her holiday in early 1977. This finally destroyed her faith in dieting, and led to the total rejection of dietary control and consequent weight gain. Her faith in diet was temporarily restored in August 1978, but it failed again about 10 months later. All this is obvious when the entire history is displayed, as in Figure 5.2, but an investigator trying to reconstruct the history of grade II obesity from this particular patient would have gleaned many different stories depending on the stage at which the investigation was made.

The disabilities and health risks associated with grade II obesity change considerably as we pass from the boundary with grade I ($W/H^2 = 30$) to the boundary with grade III ($W/H^2 = 40$). The controversy about the association of obesity with excess mortality concerns grade I, not grade II: once $W/H^2 = 30$ has been exceeded there is no doubt that mortality increases in both sexes. The life insurance data (Seltzer 1966) show an excess mortality among men of about 20% at $W/H^2 = 30$, increasing to about 100% excess mortality at $W/H^2 = 35$. Above this range life insurance data are scanty, since such people find it difficult to obtain insurance. The study of Cochrane et al (1980) on women show a similar trend of mortality with obesity index: when the women were divided into thirds by an index <25, 25–30, or <30 (ie. grades 0, I and II) the percentage deaths from all causes over a 20 year follow-up were 41, 51 and 61 in the three weight groups. Deaths from ischaemic heart disease were 8, 16 and 24 in the three weight groups. Data from the Framingham study (Gordon and Kannel 1973), and from the American Cancer Study (Lew and Garfinkel 1979) indicate similar trends in mortality with overweight in both sexes. The most important study which supports a contrary conclusion is that of Keys et al (1972). They made a very large study of the five-year incidence of coronary heart disease in men aged 40–59 at entry to the study. However the criterion of obesity was $W/H^2 > 27$, so the 'non-obese' were all grade 0 and part of grade I, while 'obese' were the upper part of grade I and higher. It has been shown in the Chicago Peoples' Gas Company study (Dyer et al 1975) and in the Framingham study (Sorlie et al 1980) that mortality tends to increase at very low weights: the weight-versus-mortality curve is U-shaped. Thus the failure of the Keys study to show much difference in coronary heart disease above and below $W/H^2 = 27$ is not evidence against an increased mortality at $W/H^2 > 30$.

Information about the cause of the excess mortality in grade II obesity is not easily extracted from life insurance data, since such people are often refused insurance. However data from slimming clubs provides some clues, since most such clubs have about 40% of their membership in the grade II weight range. The report of Rimm et al (1975) concerns the replies of 73,522 women who were members of the TOPS club to the question: 'Has a doctor ever said that you had . . . ?', where the blank is filled by the name of the disease. It is by no means certain that a 'yes' reply means that a doctor had made that diagnosis, or that if he did the diagnosis was correct. However the answers indicate that the grade II obese women were 4.5 times more likely than grade 0 women to say that a diagnosis of diabetes had been made, and 3.3 times more likely to have been diagnosed as hypertensive.

Reported gall bladder disease and gout was twice as common, and there was also a significantly ($P<0.001$) greater frequency of thyroid disease, heart disease, arthritis and jaundice. The diagnosis of thyroid disease must be viewed with some scepticism, since this diagnosis is often suspected, but seldom found, in obese patients.

The conclusions based on self-reported diagnosis agree well with the prevalence of disease associated with overweight in the American Cancer Society study (Lew and Garfinkel 1979). Among people in the grade II obesity category (ie. 115–154% of index weight for men, and 136–182% for women) the major factor in the increased mortality was coronary disease, which was about twice as common in both sexes in grade II obese people compared with those of average weight. The prevalence of diabetes was even more increased in overweight men and women (five to eight-fold), but this was less often the certified cause of death. Cancer, digestive diseases and cerebrovascular diseases were all increased in the overweight groups.

All this shows that excess mortality and morbidity is associated with excess weight, but it does not prove that the excess weight is the cause. More to the point, as Mann (1974) comments, 'It is of the utmost importance to know whether a clinical trial of weight reduction would either correct or prevent these health impairments'. This is a very reasonable suggestion, but very difficult to follow. Ideally we should take a group of obese people and randomly assign one half to a programme of weight reduction while the other half serves as a control. This ideal is unattainable for several reasons. First, we do not know how to reduce overweight, or how to prevent obesity, in a sufficiently large group of people to make analysis of the trial valid. Second, if we did have this capacity it would be unethical to have an untreated control group, since the circumstantial evidence that the untreated group would be at a disadvantage is too strong.

The circumstantial evidence that weight loss is beneficial to obese patients is reviewed in Chapter 2. In some cases the benefit is obvious quite quickly: for example to the obese diabetic or the obese middle-aged woman with osteoarthritic knees. Longer-term effects on mortality are more difficult to demonstrate, but certainly the life insurance data show that people who were refused insurance at normal premiums on account of obesity, and who subsequently attain normal weight, have a mortality record comparable to that of people who were never overweight. This is experience based on 2300 people, and it is difficult to escape the conclusion that the excess risk associated with overweight is reversible by weight loss (Dublin 1953).

The most potent agent to achieve this weight loss is a low-energy diet, which is considered in the next section.

PRINCIPLES OF LOW-ENERGY DIETS

A low-energy, or reducing, diet is the principal method used in the treatment of obesity. The diet should have the following characteristics:
1 It must not supply the energy requirements of the patient. This is an essential and inescapable characteristic of any reducing diet, since if it does supply the patient's energy requirements there is no reason why the patient's own energy stores (mainly fat) should be used up.
2 It should meet requirements for nutrients other than energy.
3 It should be acceptable to the patient. This is obviously a desirable characteristic, but one on which some compromise will be necessary. Clearly, a low-energy diet cannot have been the one which an obese patient would have consumed from choice, since otherwise the patient would not be obese. Within limitations, however, it is important to consider matters of taste, and social, economic and religious factors, so as to devise a diet which is as far as possible acceptable to the patient.
4 The diet should not impair health or well-being in other ways. For example, diets very low in fibre may cause constipation.

Books on the treatment of obesity tend to become suddenly vague and evasive when they come to deal with the real point of the problem. Let it be clearly stated here that the effectiveness of a reducing diet depends on the food which the obese patient refrains from eating. Patients are all too willing to believe that they are adhering faithfully to the prescribed diet if they eat heroic quantities of, say, lettuce, but neither lettuce nor any other food has the power to reduce fat stores. In order to put the principles of reducing diets into practice it is necessary to consider the energy, and other nutrients, provided by foods.

CONTRIBUTION OF FOOD GROUPS TO ENERGY INTAKE

From time to time governmental agencies try to find out what people are eating. It is a difficult task, involving much labour, and the results of such surveys are always open to criticism. In the United States the Department of Health, Education and Welfare mounted a huge survey in the period 1971–74. A probability sample of the U.S. population aged 1–74 years was examined, and the data concerning dietary intake are published in a paperback volume which weighs 1.5 kg (U.S. Department of Health, Education and Welfare 1979). Unfortunately the data are based on a dietary interview, consisting of a food frequency questionnaire and a recall of food consumption over a 24 hour period. This system is known to be very unreliable (Marr 1971), and it is hard to believe the published results. For example, about 10% of adult women are said to have a daily energy intake less than 700 kcal

(3 MJ) per day. No doubt this number of women recalled (or told the interviewer that they recalled) eating so little on the previous day, but it is highly improbable that this result was correct.

An alternative system by which it is possible to estimate what people are eating is the National Food Survey of domestic food consumption, (Ministry of Agriculture, Fisheries and Food 1978) in the U.K. Throughout the year (apart from a break at Christmas time, and during general election campaigns) individual private households keep a record of food consumed in the home. This source of data is open to criticism, since it provides no information about the intake of

Table 5.1 Approximate values for the composition of food groups, and their contribution to the average diet in the U.K. For values for individual food items see Appendix 2

Food group	Composition per 100 g		Protein energy as % total energy	Average consumption (g/day/ person)	Contribution of food group to total dietary intake			
	Protein (g)	Energy (kcal)			Protein (g)	(%)	Energy (kcal)	(%)
Meat	24	250	38	140	34	42	350	16
Eggs	12	150	32	30	4	5	45	2
Fish	20	160	50	17	3	4	27	1
Milk	3.3	65	20	360	12	15	234	10
Cream	2	330	—	15	—	—	50	2
Cheese	25	300	33	18	5	6	54	2
Bread	8	230	14	140	11	13	322	15
Other cereals	7	300	9	80	6	7	240	11
Butter	—	740	—	20	—	—	148	7
Margarine	—	730	—	10	—	—	73	3
Fats and oils	—	890	—	10	—	—	89	4
Sugar	—	400	—	50	—	—	200	9
Preserves	—	260	—	10	—	—	26	1
Potatoes	2	80	10	180	4	5	144	6
Fresh veg.	1	10	40	60	1	1	6	—
Canned & root vegetables	1	25	16	100	1	1	25	1
Fruit	0.6	50	9	90	1	1	45	2
Nuts	15	500	12	—	—	—	—	—
Other (incl. alcohol)							172	8
Totals				1330	82	100	2250	100

Where contribution is negligibly small this is indicated by —.

individual people within the household, nor does it record intake of alcoholic drinks, or chocolate or sugar confectionery. However, it is probably the best source from which a reliable estimate of average food intake can be derived.

To find out the contribution of a given weight of foodstuff to intake of energy, or any other nutrient, it is necessary to consult Food Tables, such as those of Paul and Southgate (1978). By combining these two reference sources it is possible to compile a picture of the Average British Diet: this is set out in Table 5.1. The average British person eats about 1330 g of food per day, which supplies about 2250 kcal (9.4 MJ) and about 82 g of protein. Obviously this average figure is made up from innumerable different individual patterns, but for the purposes of this discussion let us assume that we have an obese patient whose diet happens to correspond to the population average.

Applying the first principle of low-energy diets, it is necessary to reduce energy intake below requirements. This could be achieved simply by halving the amount of each item of food, so the diet would weigh half as much, and would supply 1125 kcal (4.7 MJ) and 41 g of protein, and half the previous amount of vitamins and minerals. This is not the best solution. In Figure 5.3 the data from Table 5.1 are presented graphically. The area assigned to each food group is in proportion to the contribution of that food group to total energy intake. Within the food group sector the shaded area indicates the proportion of energy provided by protein. It is clear in this example that about half of the dietary protein comes from meat, fish and eggs,

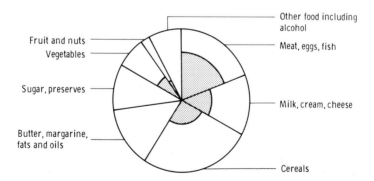

Fig. 5.3 Contribution of food groups to energy and protein intake in an average household in the U.K. The total area of the circle indicates total energy intake, and the area of the segments indicates the contribution of the food group to that total. The shaded area within the segments indicates the contribution of the food groups to protein intake. For numerical data on which diagram is based see Table 5.1

and of the remainder the great majority comes from dairy produce or cereal. These two food groups provide roughly equal amounts of protein, because, although cereal has a lower concentration of protein than milk or cheese, it is consumed in greater quantity. Vegetables, fruit and nuts all have a significant protein content, but as they contribute so little to the energy intake their contribution to protein intake is correspondingly small. Butter, margarine, cooking fats and oils, sugar, preserves, soft drinks, confectionery and alcoholic drinks make a negligible contribution to protein intake.

Figure 5.4 is constructed in a similar manner, and shows the energy sources of an individual whose requirements would have been met by the 'average' diet, shown in Figure 5.3, but who is only eating half-quantities of each foodstuff. The energy sources derived from the diet are shown on the right-hand half of the diagram, and that derived from body energy stores is shown on the left. When illustrated in this way it is clear that a 'half-quantity' diet is in effect a rather low-protein, high-fat diet. This diet has two advantages and three disadvantages. Its good points are that it is a true low-energy diet which will cause long-term fat loss, and also it is economical, since the cost of food will be roughly halved. However there are disadvantages to be set against these merits: the first and most important is that it is very unlikely to be acceptable to the patient in the long term. This chapter is concerned with the treatment of Grade II obesity, and from the arguments reviewed in

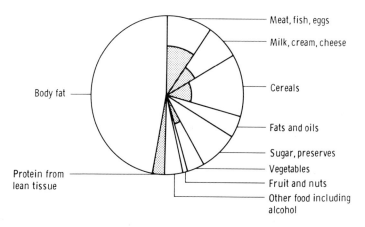

Fig. 5.4 Energy sources for a person consuming half the average diet. The contribution of each food group in Figure 5.3 has been halved, so the diet now only supplies half the energy requirements, the other half is provided by body fat and protein from lean tissue

Chapter 2, pp. 11–12, such a patient will need to keep to the diet for many months to achieve desirable weight. Among the factors regulating energy intake (see Chapter 3, pp. 47–48) habit is very important. If a person has been accustomed to having a boiled egg for breakfast it is improbable that he will take kindly to having half a boiled egg instead. Thus the diet is impractical for the treatment of severe obesity, where a considerable energy deficit is required over a long time, although a policy of reducing portion sizes by, say, 20% is quite effective in controlling minor degrees of obesity, which are discussed in later chapters.

There are two other objections to the 'half-quantity' diet, even if it were acceptable. There is at least a theoretical danger that it will be deficient in nutrients such as iron or water-soluble vitamins, and (for those who are concerned about the matter) it has a high ratio of saturated to non-saturated fat, since almost half of the energy is derived from animal fat, namely that of the patient, in addition to the fat in the diet. These points are discussed more fully in the next section. Finally the diet is not very efficient from the viewpoint of sparing the lean tissue of the patient. The importance of this was discussed in the section on starvation (Chapter 4, p. 79).

Two alternative diets which retain most of the advantages of the 'half-quantity' diet, but to some extent escape its disadvantages, are shown in Table 5.2. The simplest version is the milk diet: the sole energy source is 1800 ml (3 pints) of ordinary whole liquid milk daily. This shares with the 'half-quantity' diet the merits that it is low in energy and cheap. It is rather more acceptable than the half-quantity diet, since, if a person adopts such a diet, their habits concerning portion sizes for other foods are irrelevant. It also provides quite a high protein intake (59g) which has a greater protein-sparing effect than the 41 g which come with the half-quantity diet. The outstanding disadvantages of the milk diet are that it is totally devoid of dietary fibre, and deficient in iron and many vitamins. These deficiencies can be made good by supplying a daily tablet of ferrous sulphate and a multivitamin mixture. Finally, the milk diet is not tolerated by patients with deficiency of intestinal lactase, which is a common situation in adult Negro people. This diet will not be discussed further here, since its use is reviewed in Chapter 4.

The 'conventional' reducing diet shown in Table 5.2 is an attempt to obtain a better compromise. The energy sources for a person on the milk diet, and on this 'conventional' diet are shown in Figures 5.5 and 5.6 respectively. The diets are similar in providing slightly more than half the estimated requirements of our hypothetical average obese patient, and are similar in their effects on tissue loss: in each case the

Table 5.2 Comparison of energy sources of an average person on (a) an average diet, (b) 1800 ml of milk, and (c) a 'conventional' reducing diet

Food group	Average diet (a)			1800 milk (b)			'Conventional' diet (c)		
	Wt (g)	Prot. (g)	Energy (kcal)	Wt (g)	Prot. (g)	Energy (kcal)	Wt. (g)	Prot. (g)	Energy (kcal)
Meat	140	34	350	—	—	—	100	24	250
Eggs	30	4	45	—	—	—	30	4	45
Fish	17	3	27	—	—	—	20	4	32
Milk	360	12	234	1800	59	1170	300	10	195
Cream	15	—	50	—	—	—	—	—	—
Cheese	18	5	54	—	—	—	20	5	60
Bread	140	11	322	—	—	—	100	8	230
Other cereals	80	6	240	—	—	—	—	—	—
Butter	20	—	148	—	—	—	10	—	74
Margarine	10	—	73	—	—	—	—	—	—
Fats and oils	10	—	89	—	—	—	—	—	—
Sugar	50	—	200	—	—	—	—	—	—
Preserves	10	—	26	—	—	—	—	—	—
Potatoes	180	4	144	—	—	—	200	4	160
Fresh veg.	60	1	6	—	—	—	200	2	20
Canned & root vegetables	100	1	25	—	—	—	100	1	25
Fruit & nuts	90	1	45	—	—	—	200	2	100
Other (incl. alcohol)			172	—	—	—	—	—	—
Totals	1330	82	2250	1800	59	1170	1280	64	1191
Tissue lost									
Lean tissue	—	—	—	40	8	32	40	8	32
Fatty tissue	—	—	—	131	—	1048	128	—	1027
		82	2250		67	2250		72	2250

patient would lose about 8 g of tissue protein, which is equivalent to about 40 g of lean tissue, assuming that the lean tissue is about 20% protein. The remainder of the energy deficit is drawn from fatty tissue. When allowance is made for the water content of adipose tissue the yield of energy from 1 kg of adipose tissue is about 7500 kcal (31 MJ). (If adipose tissue was pure fat it would have an energy equivalent of 9000 kcal (38 MJ) per kg). Thus in the long term both diets would be expected to produce a rate of weight loss of about 170 g per day, or just over 1 kg per week. This prediction is subject to three important

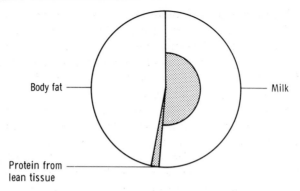

Fig. 5.5 Energy sources for a person taking 1800 ml of milk per day. Assuming energy expenditure is 2250 kcal (9.4 MJ) just over half this requirement is supplied by the milk, and the remainder is supplied by body fat and protein from lean tissue

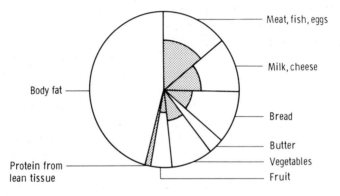

Fig. 5.6 Energy sources for a person on a 'conventional' reducing diet. The contribution of food groups has been adjusted to favour those of high protein and nutrient value, and greatly to reduce sugar, preserves and fats. The effect of body fat and protein stores is similar to that achieved by the milk diet illustrated in Figure 5.5. For numerical data on which the diagram is based see Table 5.2

qualifications: first, it assumes that the patient uses 2250 kcal (9.4 MJ) per day while taking the diet; second, it assumes that the diet is accurately observed; third, it assumes that the glycogen stores of the body are in a steady state. These assumptions are dealt with more fully on pages 123–131, when the practicalities of dietary management of obesity are considered. Since this section concerns the principles of low-energy diets we must return to considering the 'conventional' diet, and the reasons for restricting the consumption of food from some groups, while actually increasing that from other groups.

The design of the conventional reducing diet rests on several reasonable assumptions (Sebrell, 1975). The absolute requirements that it should be low in energy should be reconciled with a need to provide a high protein:energy ratio, a reasonably normal bulk, adequacy of other nutrients, and 're-education in the attitude and behaviour towards food', so the obese person comes to adopt the diet as a new way of eating for a lifetime.

It is obvious that if the diet is to have a high protein:energy ratio sugar, preserves and fats must be severely restricted, since these food groups provide energy without significant amounts of protein (see Table 5.1). In the average diet, with 82 g protein and 2250 kcal, protein provides about 14% of the total energy. The most protein-rich foods are meat, eggs, fish, milk, cheese and vegetables. It is also obvious that if the diet is to have roughly normal bulk for less-than-normal energy it must feature foods with low energy-to-weight ratios. Inspection of Table 5.1 shows that the average energy:weight ratio is about 170 kcal/100 g since 2250 kcal are provided in 1330 g of diet. The protein-containing foods with lower energy:weight ratios than this are vegetables and fruit, while meat has rather a high energy:weight ratio.

When these principles are applied the conventional reducing diet shown in Table 5.2, and in Figure 5.6 emerges. Meat is slightly restricted, since it has a high energy:weight ratio, but not omitted since it is an important protein source, and also a source of other nutrients such as iron and vitamin B_{12}. Eggs, fish, milk and cheese are included as important protein sources with reasonably low energy:weight ratios, but cream is excluded, since it does not have these desirable characteristics.

Bread is permitted in restricted quantities: it is a moderate protein source, with a moderate energy density, and it is a cheap staple food which is an important source of nutrients especially wheat fibre. A minimal allowance of 10 g of butter (or margarine) is shown in the interests of acceptability, but otherwise fats are omitted, as are sugar, preserves, and cereals (other than bread) which includes items such as cakes and biscuits.

Vegetables and fruit are the food groups in which an increased intake is advised, since these contribute to bulk and hence (perhaps) to satiety. They are also sources of Vitamin C and folate. The 'other including alcohol' group is forbidden.

Before concluding this section of the contribution of food groups to energy intake it is necessary to draw attention to the heading of Table 5.1. For purposes of this discussion it has been assumed that 'meat' provides 24 g protein and 250 kcal (1 MJ) per 100 g of edible portion. However it can be seen from the values listed in Appendix 2 that fried bacon provides about 480 kcal (1.9 MJ) per 100g, while stewed ox kidney provides only 170 kcal (0.7 MJ). The average figure of 250 kcal/100 g is a useful guide, but it depends on the type of meat and the way in which it is cooked. Within other food groups even larger variability is seen: for example cottage cheese has only a quarter of the energy:weight ratio of the high-fat cheeses. One must therefore regard with great caution statements such as 'the Weightwatchers ladies' diet provides 1295 kcal per day': such precision is unattainable even if the exact quantity of each food in the diet is known. In the construction of tables in this section I have sometimes been forced to enter values for the protein or energy value of foods to more than two significant figures, but this must not be taken to mean that corresponding accuracy is implied.

REQUIREMENTS FOR PROTEIN, VITAMINS, MINERALS AND FIBRE

Protein quality
Dietary protein is required as a source of aminoacids for tissue protein synthesis. Some proteins, such as gelatin and haemoglobin, have a low biological value, because they contain too little of some of the essential aminoacids. However mixtures of proteins can have a higher biological value than that of any component of the mixture, since one protein relatively rich in, for example, lysine, can supplement other proteins which are deficient in this aminoacid. In the older textbooks proteins were classified as 'first class' if they were of animal origin, and 'second class' if they were of vegetable origin. It is true that the meat and milk of animals usually has a good aminoacid pattern for human nutrition, since they are mixtures of many different proteins, and hence it is statistically improbable that they will be significantly deficient in an essential aminoacid. However the two examples mentioned above, haemoglobin and gelatin, are animal proteins and they certainly have no claim to be called first class nutritionally. They are specialised proteins designed to transport oxygen, or to form tough inert connective tissue respectively, and have abnormal aminoacid patterns.

The reference pattern of aminoacids against which other protein mixtures were judged was, until 1965, egg protein. This is very rich in the sulphur-containing aminoacids methionine and cystine, and consequently many dietary mixtures were pronounced deficient in these aminoacids. However recent work has shown that human aminoacid requirements are met by a lower concentration of sulphur-containing aminoacids (FAO/WHO 1973), so a new reference pattern has been set. In Table 5.3 the aminoacid pattern of the British diet,

Table 5.3 Essential aminoacid (mg/g N) in the average British diet and in milk protein, compared with the reference mixture (FAO/WHO 1973) Data for British diet from Buss and Ruck (1977)

Aminoacid	British diet	% of FAO/WHO standard	Cow's milk	% of FAO/WHO standard
Isoleucine	295	118	350	140
Leucine	498	113	640	145
Lysine	393	116	510	150
Phenylalanine	296 }	134	340 }	163
Tyrosine	214 }		280 }	
Cystine	96 }	109	60 }	109
Methionine	143 }		180 }	
Threonine	255	102	310	124
Tryptophan	79	132	90	150
Valine	351	113	460	153

based on National Food Survey data, is compared with the FAO/WHO standard (Buss and Ruck, 1977). It is evident that no essential aminoacid is limiting the biological value of this protein mixture. Similarly milk has a good aminoacid pattern, which is to be expected, since it is the sole food of infants who need to be able to synthesise protein in the process of growth.

When considering adult protein requirements, therefore, it is justifiable to disregard protein quality so long as a mixed protein source is used, such as that shown in the diets on Table 5.2. However some commercially available 'liquid protein' diets are derived from hydrolysates of collagen. It is not safe to assume that such protein sources are of high biological value.

'Recommended dietary allowances' and 'requirements'

When trying to decide if a given reducing diet is adequate in nutrients 'a good basis for adequacy is the Recommended Dietary Allowances of the National Research Council' (Sebrell 1975). If this authority is consulted the protein requirement for adult males is said to be 56 g/day, and for females 46 g/day. These are the figures revised in 1974. If the 1963 report from the same source is consulted the requirements are said to be 70 g/day for men and 58 g/day for women. In the U.K. the corresponding body is the Committee on Medical Aspects of Food Policy: in 1979 they recommended 60–84 g/day for men and 54–62 g/day for women, depending on the level of physical activity. Ten years previously the same body (DHSS, 1969) recommended 68–90 g/day for men and 55–63 g/day for women depending on physical activity, but also offered a table of 'Minimum requirements for protein' which quoted 45 g/day for men and 38 g/day for women, regardless of the level of activity. Truswell (1978) has reviewed the advice on protein requirements given by the national committees of many countries and there is great disparity between them: in the USSR certain categories of women are said to require more than 100 g/day of protein.

It should not be concluded from all this that government beaurocrats issue nonsensical recommendations without consulting the appropriate experts. The U.S. Food and Nutrition Board 'are appointed from among the leaders in the sciences related to food and nutrition . . . ' (National Academy of Sciences 1964), and no doubt the same could be said for the other national advisory committees. The trouble is that these experts are set an impossible task, and they do their best to be helpful without committing scientific perjury. Their dilemma is well stated in the Introduction to the 1979 U.K. report (DHSS 1979):

'The requirements of an individual for a nutrient is the amount needed daily to maintain health, and below which signs of deficiency might develop. Requirements differ from one individual to another and, moreover, the requirements of an individual may change with alterations in the composition and nature of the diet as a whole, because such alterations may affect the efficiency with which the nutrients are absorbed or utilized'.

The best these expert committees can do, therefore, is to calculate from the available data the average requirements of groups of healthy people, and then to add a bit more to provide a margin for safety for those with above-average requirements. It is this setting of safety margins which causes most difficulty, especially when the range of individual variation is not known.

The Recommended Dietary Allowances are a 'good basis for adequacy' when used for the purpose for which they were designed: to calculate the average requirements of a group of healthy individuals in whom it is assumed that the requirements for energy and all other nutrients are fully met. However this is certainly not the situation among obese patients on a reducing diet. We must therefore review the ways in which the special situation of a reducing diet might affect the requirements for protein and other nutrients.

Factors affecting nitrogen balance in obese patients

The only way in which it is practicable to assess the adequacy of protein in a diet is by the nitrogen balance technique. It would be impossibly tedious to feed volunteers on diets with different levels of protein until a diet was found which just failed to cause clinical evidence of protein deficiency. In regions in which protein deficiency occurs naturally it is impossible to make any accurate assessment of the diet on which the deficiency syndromes (kwashiorkor or marasmus) develop, and in any case, protein-energy malnutrition as it presents clinically is usually the result of an infection superimposed on previously marginal malnutrition, so even if the preceeding diet were accurately known it would not necessarily be sufficient in itself to cause overt disease.

However, it is not a simple matter to say a diet is adequate if it maintains nitrogen balance, since the same individual may reach nitrogen equilibrium at many differing levels of protein intake. For a given level of protein in the diet nitrogen balance is affected by the following factors:

a The time for which the diet has been consumed.

b The energy supplied by the diet, and possibly the ratio of fat to carbohydrate in the energy source.

c The nature of the diet consumed during the period immediately before the balance period.

d The fat stores of the subject.

e The characteristics of the individual subject.

Even when all the factors a to d above are held constant some subjects show greater efficiency in protein conservation than others.

From the very earliest studies of nitrogen balance (Voit 1866) it was noted that a starving dog lost nitrogen quickly for the first few days, and thereafter more slowly. It was thought that this quickly-lost component represented a 'labile protein store', and much work was done to try to identify the location and purpose of this store (Munro 1964). In the starving rat most of the 'labile' protein can be traced to the liver (Addis et al 1936), but in man this cannot be the explanation. It is now recognised that almost all body protein is in dynamic equilibrium: it is constantly catabolised and resynthesised at a rate of about 300 g/day in a normal adult. During starvation the rate of synthesis decreases almost immediately, and the rate of catabolism also decreases after a time lag. The net effect is that urinary nitrogen losses can be well described by two exponential functions: Forbes and Drenick (1979) calculate that starving obese subjects lose about 6% of body nitrogen with a half-time of 10.6 days, and the remaining 94% is then lost with a half-time of 433 days. Non-obese subjects have a smaller labile pool of about 1% of total nitrogen which is soon lost (half-time 2.4 days), and the remaining 99% of body nitrogen is then lost with a half-time of 116 days. Thus the fat stores of the obese patient serve to delay the onset of physiologically important protein depletion. The rapid weight loss during the early stages of starvation is not solely due to loss of body protein: there is also a rapid loss of salt and water (Gilder et al 1967).

The state of knowledge about the mechanism which controls energy and protein metabolism during starvation have been well reviewed by Marliss (1978) and Cahill (1978). So many things are changing that it is difficult to dissect the causes from the consequences. During starvation thyroxine is increasingly de-iodinated from the inner ring to form the inert $3,3',5'$-triiodothyronine (rT_3) instead of the active $3,5,3'$-triiodothyronine (T_3) which is formed when the outer, phenolic ring is deiodinated (Vagenakis et al 1975). Quite small quantities of carbohydrate given to the fasting subject reverse the process and cause a restoration of the T_3 concentration and a decrease in rT_3 (Azizi 1978, Burman et al 1979). The work of Vignati et al (1978) suggests that the decrease in T_3 with starvation is directly related to the conservation of protein. They gave a small dose of T_3 to subjects who had fasted for 20 days and showed that there was a significant increase in the urinary nitrogen loss, so by restoring the serum T_3 concentration to the prefasting level they reversed the adaptive response which normally spares protein during prolonged starvation.

Ketosis and the 'protein-sparing modified fast'

Bistrian (1978) recently extolled the special qualities of a diet consisting solely of 1.5 g of meat, fish or fowl protein per kg ideal body weight. He advises supplementation with a vitamin mixture, 5 g NaCl, 800 mg Ca, and potassium bicarbonate and citrate. By eliminating carbohydrate hunger is ameliorated, and the ketosis which results from this regimen is said to be important to the protein-sparing action of the diet, hence the term 'protein-sparing modified fast'. A physiological explanation for the protein-sparing effect of ketosis is given by Flatt and Blackburn (1974): they say that administration of glucose stimulates the release of insulin, insulin inhibits lipolysis, and hence the fat stores of the body are not used to make good the energy deficit caused by the low-energy diet unless carbohydrate is avoided. Thus adding carbohydrate to a reducing diet spares endogenous fat and, since the energy deficit must be met somehow, leads to increased loss of body protein, which is the only available fuel.

If the argument stated above is sound then a high-protein, very-low-carbohydrate diet is the logical way to treat obesity. However there are considerable doubts about the validity of the argument, the results actually obtained with this type of diet, and the possible hazards associated with it. Mann (1977) observes that a safe and comfortable way to lose excessive body fat is the Holy Grail of Western medicine but he regards the protein-sparing fast as a hypothesis ripe for testing, rather than the culmination of a dedicated search. The American Dietetic Association (1978) issues a warning of the dangers of adopting such a diet without strict medical supervision. One of the tantalising properties of the Holy Grail was that it disappeared from sight if approached by any person who was not of perfect purity: in similar fashion the protein-sparing effects of ketosis vanish if subjected to sceptical review. Since the relevant literature is complex and contradictory an attempt has been made to provide a synopsis in Table 5.4. Only those studies have been considered in which nitrogen balance has been measured in a metabolic ward: it is impossible to draw conclusions from outpatient studies, even when patients say they have adhered accurately to the diet. Carey et al (1963), having failed to reproduce the results reported by other investigators, say 'Contrary results can perhaps best be explained by surreptitious eating — to which the obese are notoriously liable unless carefully supervised'. In the matter of nitrogen balance on high-protein diets there is a still more subtle cause for error — if the patient does not eat the whole of the protein ration there will be an error in the balance calculation which tends to indicate greater protein sparing. Bearing in mind these reservations, the publications listed in Table 5.4 will be briefly reviewed.

Calloway and Spector (1954) analysed a very large number of studies on fit active young men to see at what level of energy and protein intake nitrogen balance was attained. These studies were of interest to people designing the most economical ration for military personnel, or for airlifting supplies to beleaguered cities. The conclusion was that protein concentrates were not a satisfactory substitute for an adequate energy supply, and that when energy intake was inadequate there was a limit to the amount of dietary protein which could be used. Figure 5.7 gives a graphical indication of the amount of protein sparing which could be achieved by adding more non-protein energy to diets with 10 g protein N, or 5g, or no protein at all. It appears from this diagram that it is impossible to achieve nitrogen equilibrium on a reducing diet. The question, therefore, was to identify the optimum point at which as much weight loss as possible was achieved with the minimum nitrogen loss.

Benoit et al (1965) compared starvation and a ketogenic diet which

Table 5.4 Synopsis of studies of nitrogen balance on low-energy diets

Authors	Date	Type of subject	N.	Diets studied	Comments
Calloway and Spector	1954	Active, non-obese young men, acute experiments, less than 14 days	646	Review of wide range of energy and N intake	Concluded: 'When caloric intake 1000 kcal, 3 gN will produce as much protein sparing as higher quantities of nitrogen.'
Benoit et al	1965	Obese naval personnel	7	Starvation & ketogenic (7.3 g N, 1000 kcal) with crossover design 10 day study periods	Concluded ketogenic diet was protein sparing: N loss with starvation 14.6 g/d, with ketogenic diet only 5.3 gN/d.
Bollinger et al	1966	Obese patients	12	Starvation & 40 g egg albumin for 8–14 days	Average N loss on starvation 7.4 g/d but with egg albumin *following* starvation only 2.4 g/d.
Apfelbaum et al	1967	Obese patients	12	Starvation, or protein supplement of 4.4 or 8.8 g N. 5 day study periods	Results reported on only 9 of 12 subjects. N balance achieved with 8.8 g N *following* starvation. No statistical analysis given.
Hood et al	1970	Obese women	4	1000 kcal diets with 3, 6, 12, 25, or 50% carbohydrate. Latin square, 8 d periods	N balance better with high carbohydrate than low carbohydrate diets, despite lower N content with high carbohydrate.
Blackburn et al	1973	Obese patients Surgical patients	8 10	Starvation vs 1 g. protein/kg. 90 g aminoacids for surgical patients	N loss on starvation 'some 6 g/d' but with meat supplement it was 'significantly reduced'. Data sparse & difficult to evaluate.

Table 5.4 continued

Authors	Date	Type of subject	N.	Diets studied	Comments
Jourdan et al	1974	Obese women	6	4 energy levels with 0, 3 or 12 g N. Sequential design without crossover	Meticulous balance technique: faecal and skin loss constant at about 2 g and 0.2 g/d respectively. N equilib. on 12 g N *following* protein-free diet.
Baird et al	1974	Obese patients	5	800 kcal, 60 g protein 900 kcal, 40 g aminoacids starvation various aminoacid & carbohydrate mixtures	Conclude: 'Optimum formulation 15 g aminoacids or egg albumin with 30–45 g carbohydrate' (in order to abolish ketosis). This diet *followed* starvation.
Bistrian et al	1975	Obese patients with infections	4	0.8–1.0 g protein/kg as lean beef	'In six infectious episodes there was no change in urinary N.' but balance data impossible to evaluate.
Jeeheebhoy	1976	Surgical patients on parenteral nutrition		0–2 g protein/kg	N balance depends on N and energy intake (cf. Calloway & Spector 1954) added carbohydrate spares protein
Yang & van Itallie	1976	Obese men	6	50 d protocol starvation, ketogenic or mixed diet: 800 kcal, 50 g protein 10 d balance periods	N loss on starvation 8.06 g/d sig. greater than ketogenic (2.86 g/d) or mixed (1.57 g/d), but no N sparing attributable to ketosis.
Apfelbaum	1976	Healthy obese women	21	55 g protein for 3 weeks	Balance negative first week, but by end of third week deficit restored. Balance more positive in younger patients. Few technical details.

Table 5.4 continued

Authors	Date	Type of subject	N.	Diets studied	Comments
Howard & Baird	1977	Obese patients	34	Starvation 15–25 g protein 20–40 g carbohydrate 180–320 kcal	N balance after 4 weeks on 25 g protein & 40 g carbohydrate, positive balance reported in 8th week.
Bistrian et al	1977a	Mildly obese young women	5	1.5 g/kg ideal body weight protein, starvation, & protein with energy	Conclude: 'After a deficit in lean body mass is produced, protein anabolism can be achieved with protein sparing modified fast.'
Bistrian et al	1977b	Prader–Willi	4	1.4–2.1 g protein/kg ideal body weight	Report consistently positive N balance throughout. N content of meat estimated from food tables.
Marliss et al	1978	Obese, non-diabetic	18	82.5 g protein, with or without previous starvation	N loss initially, but not after 12–21 days. Positive balance *after* starvation. Balance not explained by changes in insulin levels.
Howard et al	1978	Obese patients	21	31 g protein 44 g carbohydrate 320 kcal	Nitrogen balance attained in 4–6 weeks.
Wilson & Lamberts	1979	Obese patients	11	31 g protein 44 g carbohydrate 320 kcal	N loss decreased steadily with time, but still slightly negative (−1.3 g/d) after 4 weeks.
DeHaven et al	1980	Obese patients	7	100 g turkey protein, 50 g turkey protein & 50 g carbohydrate. 25–40 day balance periods, crossover design	N balance improved with time on both types of diet, and equilibrium reached by 4th week. No difference between diets in protein sparing.

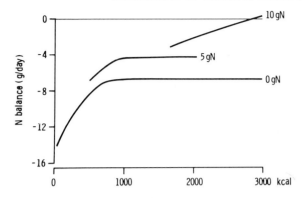

Fig. 5.7 Nitrogen balance at different levels of energy intake: acute studies in active young men, reviewed by Calloway and Spector (1954). On total starvation about 14 g N per day is lost. As the energy content of a protein-free diet is increased the nitrogen loss is decreased, but maximum protein-sparing is achieved at about 800 kcal (3.4 MJ) per day. With higher protein intakes more protein-sparing can be achieved by higher energy intakes. These results do not apply to subjects adapted to long-term low-energy diets

provided 7.3 gN (45 g protein) and 1000 kcal (4.2 MJ). Each diet was given for 10 days, and the sequence of diet periods and starvation periods was alternated to balance out the effect of adaptation with time. The observed N loss agrees well with that indicated by Figure 5.7. Bolinger et al (1966) gave 40 g of egg albumin to obese patients after they had undergone a period of total starvation: the design did not compensate for adaptation with time. The observed loss of N was less than that found either by Calloway and Spector, or by Benoit et al, and again the protein sparing effect is seen, but nitrogen balance is not achieved.

The first investigator to claim positive nitrogen balance with a protein-sparing modified fast was Apfelbaum et al (1967). The paper must be regarded with some reserve, since the results published are those of only 9 of the 12 subjects investigated, and it is not clear why the others were omitted. This paper showed that it was possible to obtain nitrogen balance by giving 55 g pure protein to patients who had previously been starved.

Thus far, the diets which had been tested were all ketogenic, and it had been shown that they improved nitrogen balance compared with total starvation. The crucial test of the role of ketosis in this protein-sparing action was to compare isoenergetic diets containing different amounts of carbohydrate. This was done by Hood et al (1970) who tested diets with 3, 6, 12, 25 or 50% of energy provided by carbohydrate, the total energy in each case being 1000 kcal (4.2 MJ).

An appropriate Latin square design was used and each balance period was 8 days. Nitrogen equilibrium was not attained in any of the balance periods, but N loss was smaller with diets with a high carbohydrate content than with the ketogenic 3% carbohydrate diet. This study argues against ketosis in itself having a protein-sparing action.

Blackburn et al (1973) measured urinary nitrogen loss in obese patients and surgical patients, and noted that a diet of meat for obese patients, or aminoacid infusions in surgical patients, reduced loss of lean tissue compared with starvation. However the protocol is not clearly stated, and the balance technique is not described, so it is not possible to make a critical evaluation of this report. Jourdan et al (1974) report a very careful study in which N losses (including dermal losses) were carefully measured. They convincingly showed that subjects who were changed from starvation to a diet which supplied half the energy requirement with 12 gN (75 g protein) went into nitrogen balance.

Meanwhile another school took the view that ketosis was a thing to be avoided, and designed diets with enough carbohydrate to eliminate ketosis. Baird et al (1974) after trying many diets sequentially concluded that the 'optimum formulation is 15 g of aminoacid or egg albumin (2.4 g N) with 30 to 45 g carbohydrate'. With this they achieved N balance, but only on well-adapted patients who had previously been starved. The results of Jeejeebhoy (1976) show that in surgical patients on parenteral nutrition carbohydrate added to aminoacid infusions improves nitrogen balance, whereas if ketosis promoted protein sparing this result would not be expected. Yang and van Itallie (1976) made a direct test of the ketosis theory by making a comparison of nitrogen balance on ketogenic or non-ketogenic 800 kcal (3.4 MJ) diets, or starvation, with the appropriate crossover design. Both diets were protein-sparing by comparison with starvation, but there was no advantage to the ketogenic diet.

Apfelbaum (1976) broke new ground by reporting that with his 'proteic' diet consisting of 55 g protein (with vitamin and mineral supplements) although there was nitrogen loss in the first week, this was recouped by the end of the third week on the diet. The publications since that time, which are listed in Table 5.4., note that nitrogen balance is attained after a few weeks, or after a period of nitrogen loss. The sole exception is the paper of Bistrian et al (1977b), which reports nitrogen balance from the first day of a diet of meat given to 4 patients with Prader-Willi syndrome. The protein content of the meat was estimated from food tables, and it is not clear how the authors knew that their subjects did in fact consume the large quantities prescribed. If (as seems likely from the nature of Prader-

Willi patients) they were not completely compliant in this matter the apparent positive nitrogen balance may well be spurious. Readers who have no personal experience of metabolic balance studies may think that too much fuss is being made about details of technique, but unless great care is taken to measure both nitrogen intake and output the results of such studies are worthless. This point is illustrated in Figure 5.8, which shows the weekly nitrogen balance of five women fed a conventional reducing diet (850 kcal, 3.55 MJ, with 45 g protein) for six weeks. At least the intended intake was 45 g protein per day, but if uneaten food is carefully weighed back it can be seen that during some weeks some patients ate significantly less than the diet which was offered. If the nitrogen balance had been calculated on the assumption that all the food offered had been eaten the result would have been an apparent positive balance.

Figure 5.8 illustrates some other points of importance in the interpretation of nitrogen balance results. First, there is considerable variability between individuals, and from week to week in the same individual, when kept on exactly the same diet. There is a strong trend towards more efficient nitrogen conservation with time, as many of the publications listed in Table 5.4 have noted, but an individual may be in positive balance one week, in negative balance the next week, and return to positive balance the week after that. Of the five patients studied (Durrant et al 1980) the one who behaved in the most regular fashion concerning nitrogen balance was patient 2, who was post-

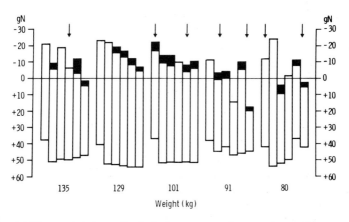

Fig. 5.8 Nitrogen balance studies in 5 obese women who were given a diet supplying 3.55 MJ per day for 6 consecutive weeks (data of Durrant et al 1980). Weekly N intake is plotted below the line, and N output in urine (open columns) and faeces (solid columns) is plotted upward. Arrows indicate the start of a menstrual period. Note the very small contribution of faecal nitrogen to total N loss, and the irregularity of N balance from week to week in several subjects

menopausal. The other patients all had one or two menstrual periods during the study, but it is difficult to explain the irregularities of nitrogen balance in relation to any particular phase of the menstrual cycle. Figure 5.9 shows the mean values ($\pm$ 1 S.D.) for nitrogen balance, weight loss, and the ratio of nitrogen loss to weight loss in the five women who were also the subjects in Figure 5.8. Just as there is a trend to diminishing nitrogen loss with time there is a trend towards diminishing weight loss, but the former effect is stronger than the latter, so the ratio of nitrogen to weight loss falls also. In this particular group of patients the average nitrogen loss in the sixth week was zero, but this mean value conceals the fact that one of the five was losing nearly 20 gN in the sixth week, while another was gaining about 10 gN in the sixth week.

During starvation subjects with large fat stores conserve nitrogen better than lean subjects (Forbes and Drenick 1979, van Itallie and Yang 1977). This factor helps to explain why the reported nitrogen balance in obese patients on low-energy diets is better than that which Calloway and Spector (1954) found in their active young men.

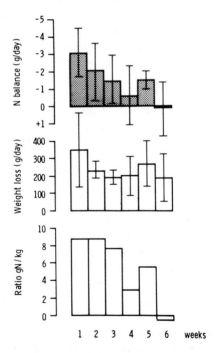

Fig. 5.9 Average values for nitrogen balance in the subjects shown in Fig 5.8. Note that both N loss and weight loss decrease with successive weeks on the low-energy diet, and the group on average was in N balance by the sixth week

To summarise, therefore: the statement that ketosis is important for protein sparing (Bistrian 1978, Flatt and Blackburn 1974) is not supported by acceptable evidence, and it is contrary to the evidence provided by studies such as that of Yang and van Itallie (1976), and Marliss et al (1978). It is probably true that a diet with a high protein content is associated with a smaller loss of lean tissue in the early stages than in an isoenergetic diet with a lower protein content. To what extent this difference matters in the long run is hard to say, since metabolic balance studies over many months are too tedious to attempt, and anyway it would be difficult to design a protocol which adequately allowed for the adaptive changes which occur in subjects on low-energy diets of any kind for long periods. We can infer from the report of Kempner et al (1975) that even a low-energy, low-protein diet is not disastrous in the long run. They report some 106 patients who lost at least 45 kg on a rice diet which provides less than 1000 kcal per day and probably less than 30 g of protein: the publication contains the astonishing statement: 'The use of carbohydrate as a caloric source takes advantage of its protein-sparing effects . . . '. No evidence for the statement is given, but the fact that patients lost weight and survived on the diet which seems ill-suited to protein conservation implies that probably obese people can adapt to almost anything short of starvation if they are given long enough to do so.

Requirements for vitamins and minerals

The recommended dietary allowances for vitamins and minerals for adult women are listed in Table 5.5. It can be seen that there is some difference between the allowances for the U.S. and the U.K. and that the U.S. 1974 report contained allowances for many vitamins and minerals for which other committees had declined to estimate requirements.

It is very difficult to provide the recommended intake of iron with any reasonable selection of food: the Weight watchers' ladies diet includes as much iron-rich food as possible, but still only provides 14 mg, rather than the recommended 18 mg (Sebrell 1975). It probably does not matter much, since the efficiency with which iron is absorbed from the gut increases with iron deficiency. In practice vitamin or mineral deficiencies occur as a result of factors other than dietary deficiency: for example the anti-folate action of anticonvulsant drugs, the potassium depletion caused by purgatives or diuretics, and mineral deficiencies due to phytate from uncooked bran inhibiting absorption from the gut.

Table 5.5   Recommended dietary allowances of vitamins and minerals for adult women: U.S. Food and Nutrition Board 1964 and 1974, and U.K. Department of Health 1969 and 1979

Nutrient	Unit	U.S. 1964	U.K. 1969	U.S. 1974	U.K. 1979
Vitamin A	μg	1000	750	800	750
Vitamin D	μg	*	2.5	10	*
Thiamine	mg	0.8	1.0	1.1	1.0
Riboflavin	mg	1.2	1.3	1.4	1.3
Niacin	mg	13	15	14	15
Folate	μg	*	*	400	300
Vitamin B_6	mg	*	*	2.0	*
Vitamin B_{12}	μg	*	*	3.0	*
Ascorbic acid	mg	70	30	45	30
Vitamin E	I.U.	*	*	12	*
Calcium	mg	800	500	800	500
Iron	mg	15	12	18	12
Phosphorus	mg	*	*	800	*
Iodine	μg	*	*	100	*
Magnesium	mg	*	*	300	*
Zinc	mg	*	*	15	*

Detection of vitamin and mineral deficiencies

Any doctor who gives dietary advice to patients should be willing and able to check that this advice is not causing significant nutritional deficiencies of vitamins or minerals. This is not easy. Most publications about weight-reduction regimens suggest that all known nutrients should be given at a level to meet the current dietary allowances, and probably say that 'close monitoring of clinical, haematological and biochemical parameters is also mandatory', or words to that effect. This advice is not helpful unless some guidance is given about the likelihood of finding significant changes, and how they should be interpreted.

It is very unlikely that patients on a low-energy diet will become deficient in vitamin A or D. The amount of vitamin A stored in the liver of normal people will meet requirements for many months or years with no dietary intake (Davidson et al 1979). If deficiency occurs the first and most sensitive sign is lessened ability to see in the dark: with severe deficiency in protein-depleted children there is loss of shininess of the conjunctiva which progresses to xerophthalmia, keratomalacia, and destruction of the cornea. It is doubtful if there is any dietary requirement for vitamin D in adults who have normal exposure to sunlight. Since vitamins A and D are toxic in overdose it is important that large supplements of these vitamins should not be prescribed to dieting patients unless there is good evidence of deficiency. If such evidence is found it is more likely that the cause is malabsorption of fat from the gut, or interference with the metabolism of the vitamin by some drug, rather than true dietary deficiency.

Thiamine deficiency is also an improbable diagnosis in a patient on a reducing diet, since thiamine requirements are linked to energy intake (Sauberlich et al 1979). Most commonly it is seen when alcohol provides a large part of the energy intake. The stores in the body of this vitamin are small, so biochemical changes are seen after only 14 days on a high-carbohydrate thiamine-free diet (Sauberlich et al 1979). The specific test of deficiency is to measure the transketolase activity of red cells with and without the addition of thiamine pyrophosphate: an increase of activity of more than 25% indicates deficiency. Fortunately the vitamin is not toxic, since if excess is given it is rapidly cleared in the urine.

Riboflavin deficiency causes angular stomatitis and vascularisation of the cornea, but these signs are not diagnostic of riboflavin deficiency. If in doubt it is possible to try the effect of vitamin supplement (5 mg three times per day) since there are no reported toxic effects at this dosage.

Niacin, or nicotinic acid, is the pellagra-preventing factor. It can be synthesised from tryptophan: it is calculated that 60 mg of tryptophan is equivalent to one mg of niacin. If the urinary excretion of N'-methylnicotinamide is less than 1.6 mg/g urinary creatinine this suggests deficient intake or absorption.

It is difficult to make accurate measurements of the available folate in diets, hence the reticence of committees to state dietary requirements. Folate deficiency causes megaloblastic anaemia, but treatment with folic acid must not be given unless it is established that the anaemia is not due to B_{12} deficiency, or it may worsen the neurological features of Addisonian anaemia. Deficiency of folate is indicated by a low red cell folate concentration. If deficiency is found this may be due to the effect of drugs such as anticonvulsants, rather than dietary deficiency, and if large amounts of folate are given this may reduce the effectiveness of the anticonvulsant treatment.

Vitamin B_{12} deficiency occurs in people who cannot absorb the vitamin, or sometimes in those who totally avoid food of animal origin. Deficiency causes megaloblastic anaemia, and the diagnosis can be made from the low plasma B_{12} concentration or by the rapid haematological response when the vitamin is given.

Of all the vitamins ascorbic acid, or vitamin C, is the one required in the greatest quantity by the human species, monkeys and guinea pigs (see Table 5.5). Deficiency causes scurvy, which was an important cause of death among sailors who lived for months without fresh fruit. The clinical signs are swollen bleeding gums or petechial haemorrhage in the skin. Since the vitamin is not toxic even in vast overdose it should be given if the diagnosis is suspected rather than wait for the results of laboratory tests.

Concerning mineral status, iron deficiency is by far the most easily diagnosed, since the clinically important effect is a hypochromic anaemia. The diagnosis can be confimed by measurement of the serum iron concentration, since there are other causes of hypochromic anaemia.

Dietary deficiency of calcium, phosphorus or magnesium is very difficult to diagnose, since there is a vast reservoir of these elements in the skeleton. Indeed many publications on protein-sparing fasting regimens seem to have ignored most mineral requirements. Apfelbaum (1976), Vertes et al (1977) and Bistrian (1978) emphasise the need for potassium supplements, but do not mention any need for any of the minerals listed in Table 5.5. Concerning patients on his rice diet Kempner (1975) says 'The diet is supplemented daily with multi-vitamins to prevent any possible nutritional deficiencies', but 1000 kcal of boiled rice comes nowhere near supplying the requirements of iron, calcium or magnesium.

Requirements for dietary fibre

No expert committee has ventured to state a recommended daily intake of dietary fibre, but it could be argued that deficiency of fibre has caused more ill-health than, for example, has been caused in man by deficiency of vitamin E or zinc. Dietary fibre is an emotive subject: its proponents claim that a high-fibre diet 'can protect you from six of the most serious diseases of civilization' (Reuben, 1975). Such rather wild statements are based on associations between the prevalence of certain types of bowel disease, heart disease and cancer and the consumption of dietary fibre. Much of the evidence is anecdotal: the population of rural Africa may eat a lot of fibre and suffer little cancer, but it is necessary to show that they live to an age at which they might be expected to develop cancer before any beneficial effect can be ascribed to the fibre intake. Furthermore, the experts keep changing the definition of 'dietary fibre', which is a mixture of cellulose, hemicelluloses, lignin, pectin, gums and alginates which cannot be absorbed from the human gut (Southgate 1976). All 'roughage' does not have equal effect on bowel function: the lignified cell wall from wheat bran is particularly resistant to the action of colonic bacteria, and is the most effective type of fibre for increasing stool weight and decreasing transit time (Cummings et al 1979). This is of importance, since the proportion of cereal fibre in the diet, and also the absolute amount of fibre in the diet, has steadily declined over the past century (Southgate et al 1978).

Aspects of dietary fibre which are of importance in designing reducing diets are the capacity of fibre to promote satiety, and to lower blood lipids. These matters are discussed on pages 116 and 120 respectively. However an interesting, and so far unexplained, association between fibre intake and heart disease was reported by Morris et al (1977). Among 337 healthy middle-aged men who were followed for 10–20 years there were 45 who developed clinical coronary heart disease. When the men were divided into thirds by their intake of fibre, or of cereal fibre, the third with the lowest fibre intake contained 25 cases of coronary heart disease, while the third with the highest fibre intake had only 5 cases of coronary heart disease. It has been observed that obese patients on fibre-free supplemented fasts sometimes die of coronary heart disease (Vertes et al 1977a), and it is at least a tenable hypothesis that deficiency of cereal fibre may have increased their susceptibility to heart disease. However, it would not necessarily be a good plan to add liberal amounts of wheat bran to the diet, since quite a lot of carbohydrate in bran is absorbed, and hence is an energy source (see Appendix 2), and the phytic acid in uncooked bran may prevent the normal absorption of minerals from the gut.

HUNGER, SATIETY AND APPETITE

One of the unpleasant features about low-energy diets is that they cause hunger. Since the diet should be made as acceptable as possible to the patient it is desirable to arrange that, for a given energy intake, as little hunger as possible is caused. It has been claimed as a merit of ketogenic diets (Bistrian 1978), and non-ketogenic diets (Baird et al 1974), and high-fibre diets (Grimes and Goddard 1977) and even of total starvation (Bolinger et al 1966), that this particular type of diet causes little hunger. Such statements must be viewed with scepticism unless the authors made a serious attempt to measure hunger. Just because patients do not complain vociferously to the investigator that they are hungry this does not prove that they are not hungry.

It might be supposed that people could be relied upon to say if they were hungry so long as they were asked, but measuring hunger is not a simple matter. Even in semistarvation of severe degree reports of what the victims regard as 'hunger' are surprising. Among Jews starving to death in the Warsaw ghetto (Winick 1979) the early signs were thirst, polyuria, weight loss and a constant craving for food, but with time these diminished and were replaced by feelings of weakness, coldness, followed by exhaustion and death. In less extreme experimental semistarvation of volunteers Keys et al (1950) say

'It should be stressed that the discomfort caused by hunger pain is by no means the most important change resulting from semistarvation. In men who were unable to adhere to the diet ... the "hunger pangs" did not seem to be present in any manifestly exaggerated degree'.

To test the effect of a low-energy diet on hunger probably the most practical method is to use a rating scale with 'not at all hungry' at one end and 'the most hungry I have ever been' at the other: the subject indicates his present feeling by a mark somewhere between these two extremes. Silverstone et al (1966) using a similar method failed to detect any less hunger among 9 patients on total starvation than they had recorded from these patients on a conventional 4.2 MJ (1000 kcal) diet. Thus the claim that starvation confers some protection from the sensation of hunger has not been substantiated.

The complex factors which affect energy intake are reviewed on pages 43 to 49: in this section the effect of the composition and meal frequency of a reducing diet will be considered as it affects acceptability.

Heaton (1973) has suggested that the fibre content of the diet is an important factor in regulating energy intake, and Hunt et al (1978) suggest that the lower the energy density of the diet the slower the absorption of energy, since gastric emptying is also slower. Grimes and Goddard (1977) have shown that gastric emptying is slower after eating wholemeal bread than after eating white bread. It might be expected, therefore, that volunteers given substantial amounts of wholemeal bread would have a lower spontaneous energy intake thereafter than when they were given white bread, but Bryson et al (1979) failed to observe this effect. Although it is possible to make a plausible argument that a high fibre intake ought to restrict energy intake there is no convincing evidence that it does so (van Itallie 1978).

There is very little reliable information about the effect of different ratios of fat to carbohydrate in the diet on spontaneous energy intake.

This is an important matter, on which conflicting advice is given. Often obese patients will say that they do not eat much, but that they probably eat the 'wrong sort of food'. When asked what sort of food this is some say that fatty foods are known to be particularly fattening: the more sophisticated ones will quote evidence that high-fat diets produce obesity in rats, that fats have more energy per unit weight, and that the deposition of fat in adipose tissue is metabolically more efficient when fat is the precursor than when carbohydrate or protein is the energy source. All of this is true, but others can produce equally compelling reasons for selectively restricting carbohydrate. High carbohydrate foods are stigmatised as 'junk foods', lacking nutrients and unable to stimulate satiety; carbohydrate stimulates insulin secretion and hence hunger rather than the satiety produced by fats. An interesting attempt to find out what in fact happens to spontaneous intake when the fat:carbohydrate ratio was altered was reported by van Stratum et al (1978). A formula diet, providing 4.18 kJ (1 kcal) per g, was prepared in two recipes: formula A provided 20% of the energy as fat and 61% as carbohydrate, while formula B had the proportions reversed: in both formulae protein provided 19% of the energy. Over a period of 4 weeks 22 Trappist nuns derived most of their energy from one or other formula, with a balanced crossover design. If either fat or carbohydrate was much more satiating there should have been a significantly lower intake of one or other formula, but this was not found. There were large variations between individuals, and from day to day within individuals, but no general pattern emerges. It should be noted that the test foods were made up as drinks, and the formulae were adjusted to give equal energy density, so the results do not necessarily reflect behaviour when eating normal food.

The effect of energy density on hunger experienced by obese patients on a low-energy diet has been systematically investigated by Durrant and Mann (1977). They used two pairs of experimental diets in which the energy content and the volume were manipulated in opposite directions, as shown below:

	Energy kJ	(kcal)	Weight g	Energy density (kJ/g)
Diet A	992	237	474	2.09
Diet B	1548	370	367	4.20
Diet C	1933	462	769	2.51
Diet D	2971	710	594	5.00

Patients were fed diet A and B on one pair of days, and C and D on another pair of days, and after each pair they were asked to assess which day had been associated with the higher energy intake. If patients were chiefly influenced by the amount of food they would choose A and C; if they could detect the true energy content despite the conflicting effect of energy density they would chose B and D, and if they were unable to pick up any reliable signals from the diets the answers would be random. The study was a closed sequential design, so it terminated when 15 out of 19 patient choices were for diets B or D, since this indicated ($P<0.05$) that obese patients could correctly identify the diet with 50% more energy, even when energy density had been manipulated to give a false indication of the energy content.

From these studies, and others which are reviewed on pages 46–49, it appears that there is no modification of the fat: carbohydrate ratio, or of the energy density of a diet, which can materially enhance its ability to allay hunger, or induce satiety, relative to another diet of similar energy content. However there are two other aspects of a diet which have considerable influence on its acceptability and the amount which will be consumed. When patients in a metabolic ward are given a low energy diet as either one or five meals per day, most greatly prefer the five-meal regimen (Garrow et al 1981). Although the 'nibbling' mode of eating does not appear to affect fat loss, it does seem to cause less hunger or discomfort than 'gorging' an isoenergetic diet.

Finally, the palatability of the diet has an important effect on appetite. Yudkin (1963) makes a useful distinction between hunger and appetite: hunger is a sensation which makes you want to eat, but appetite is a sensation which makes you want to eat a particular food. Generally speaking, palatability is achieved by providing a variety of foods, and this makes biological sense, because a varied diet is less likely to be deficient in a particular nutrient than one which is based on a single staple food. It is common experience, supported by formal evidence in both experimental animals and in man (Rolls et al 1979) that satiety is specific to particular foods. We may have eaten our fill of a meat course, and be virtually unable to eat more, but appetite revives amazingly when strawberries and cream are offered. Thus spontaneous intake will be lower on a monotonous diet, since once hunger is satisfied on such a diet there is no further stimulus to appetite. The practical question is — should reducing diets be deliberately made unpalatable? A reasonable answer is that it is unwarrantable to expect obese people to keep to a diet of foods which they do not like, even in small quantities, but that it may well be helpful to restrict the variety of foods offered in the diet. Thus satiety to permitted foods might be achieved on an energy intake much lower than that which would have been required for a more varied fare. Experimental evidence shows that both obese and normal weight people do eat less if they are offered a monotonous diet (Campbell et al 1971, Cabanac and Rabe 1976). However anyone who advocates monotonous diets for use over a long period has a responsibility to ensure that it is not deficient in some essential nutrient other than energy.

THE ECONOMICS OF REDUCING DIETS

Among the many reasons which obese patients may give for not keeping to a reducing diet one is that it is too expensive: they would be quite happy to eat steak and salad all day, but cannot afford to do so. This is a point worth consideration, since food is a major item in the budget of most households.

Obviously if the patient adopts the half-quantity diet shown in Figure 5.4 (p. 93) this cannot be more expensive than a normal diet. However, if the energy previously provided by bread and other cereals, fats, sugar and preserves is obtained from meat, vegetables and fruit the cost of the diet may increase considerably. Within any food group there is a large range of cost, but in general meat, vegetables and fruit are expensive energy sources, and those food groups which do not provide significant amounts of protein are relatively cheap energy sources. Figure 5.10 was constructed by comparing the average expenditure of households on each food group with the contribution of that food group to total protein and energy intake. The ratio of total expenditure on food to total intake of energy and protein was taken as

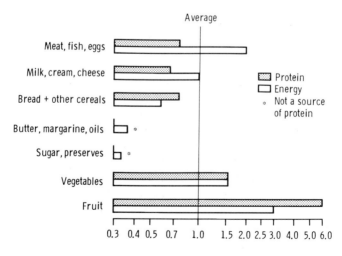

Fig. 5.10 Relative cost of protein and energy derived from different food groups. The average cost of protein and of energy in the whole diet is 1.0

the reference value 1.0. It can be seen that sugar as an energy source costs 0.33 of the average energy cost, and fats also are very cheap energy sources. However protein or energy derived from vegetables cost 1.5 times the average cost, and protein from fruit costs 6 times, and energy from fruit 3 times, that of the diet as a whole.

In the 'conventional' diet shown in Table 5.2 the food groups in which increased intake is suggested are fresh vegetables and fruit. However there are reductions in meat, cream, cereals, fats, sugar, preserves and 'other, including alcohol', so the total cost of the diet comes out slightly less than that of the normal diet.

SUGAR, FATS AND CHOLESTEROL

Experts in the United States (U.S. Select Committee on Nutrition and Human Needs 1977) and elsewhere have advised that the consumption of saturated fat and sucrose should be reduced, and that of complex carbohydrates should be increased, with a view to providing some protection against coronary heart disease. So far as reducing diets are concerned sucrose and fat intake is anyway restricted, so the only problems which occur relate to cholesterol and unsaturated fat.

In epidemiological studies of heart disease (Keys 1970) the factors most strongly linked with prevalence were blood pressure and plasma cholesterol. Should eggs (an important source of cholesterol) be excluded from low-energy diets? The answer is probably not, because dietary intake of cholesterol has little influence on the plasma cholesterol concentration (Oliver 1978). The evidence that a high intake of unsaturated fat confers benefit is very weak (McMichael 1979). Probably the most useful thing the obese person can do to reduce his liability to heart disease is to lose weight.

THE OBESE DIABETIC

Diabetes mellitus is a severe threat to the obese person. In the experience of life insurance companies death attributable to diabetes is four-times commoner in overweight people than in people of normal weight (Donald 1973). This is not a peculiarity of those who take out life insurance: the very large survey by the American Cancer Society (Lew and Garfinkel 1979) tells the story still more clearly. Among men more than 140% of average weight the total mortality rate was 1.87 times that of average weight men, but the mortality from diabetes in the overweight men was 5.19 times the mortality from diabetes in average weight men. Among women more than 140% of average weight the mortality (relative to those of average weight) was 1.89 times greater overall, but 7.90 times greater for diabetes. It appears that the combination of excess weight and impaired glucose tolerance contributes more to the risk of death from coronary heart disease than either factor alone. In the study of 18,403 civil servants in London (Fuller et al 1980) the 7½ year death rate per 1000 among those with normal glucose tolerance was 21.6 for an obesity index (W/H^2) less than 27, and 24.5 for an index over 27. Among those with impaired glucose tolerance but below 27 on the obesity scale the mortality rate was 39.8, but those who had both impaired glucose tolerance and an index above 27 the mortality rate was 56.4.

The relationship of obesity to the development of diabetes has been well reviewed by Baird (1973) and Cahill (1978). Obesity is one of several factors which determine if an individual will develop the high fasting blood sugar, glucose intolerance, glycosuria, and eventually the neuropathy, vascular and renal changes which are the crippling and life-threatening complications of diabetes. The interaction of obesity with genetic factors is shown by the greater similarity in prevalence of diabetes in monozygotic than in dizygotic twins, but even in monozygotic twins concordance is not complete (Baird 1973). In a survey of diabetic patients, their brothers and sisters, and the brothers and sisters of control patients, the percentage of diabetics in the obese sibs of diabetics was 14.9, while among thin sibs of diabetics it was only 5.8. Among the obese sibs of control patients the percentage diabetic was 7.1, while among thin sibs of control patients it was only 2.0 (Baird 1973). It appears that obesity causes an increased strain on the ability of the pancreas to secrete enough insulin to control glucose metabolism, and in those individuals with a smaller reserve capacity for insulin secretion an extra load of fat is more likely to produce overt diabetes. This is an oversimplification of a complicated relationship: Genuth (1973) has calculated that the daily secretion of insulin in the normal person is 31 units, in obese persons 114 units, in juvenile diabetics 4 units, in thin adult diabetics 14 units and in obese adult diabetics 46 units. Thus the obese adult diabetic is secreting more insulin than the normal person, but less than is required for glucose homeostasis in an obese person. The high incidence of diabetes in older obese people, reflected in the high diabetic mortality rate, suggests that the insulin-secreting cells in the obese person in the end become exhausted in their effort to supply the high demands put upon them. That this is truly an effect of the added fat load, and not merely a sign of the diabetic constitution is shown by the studies on experimental obesity by Salans et al (1974): normal men with no family history of diabetes who are rendered obese by overfeeding show the same features of glucose metabolism as are found in spontaneous obesity.

It is obvious that diminishing the load of excess fat is very important in avoiding the risk of diabetes in obese people, but the risk is often not recognised until it is a reality. Seaton and Rose (1965) noted that there was a very high default rate from weight reduction clinics (23.9% did not return after the first visit) but 'the patients least likely to default from a weight reduction clinic are those with diabetes mellitus'. However it is reasonable to suppose that if these patients had applied themselves with equal fervour to dieting before their diabetes became obvious they might have retained enough insulin-secreting capacity to escape diabetes entirely.

The principles of low-energy diets which have been set out above apply equally to the management of obese adult-onset diabetics. It must be realised that control of the diabetes by a low-energy diet, or by giving extra insulin, are not equally satisfactory lines of treatment: the thing that is wrong with the obese diabetic is the obesity, not the lack of insulin. In practice control with injected insulin is often difficult to achieve, since the patient is as resistant to exogenous insulin as to his own, and the very high doses which are required probably make it all the more difficult for the patient to keep to the low-energy diet. However there are still several points about the management of the obese diabetic on which there is no consensus: what is the ideal balance of carbohydrate to total energy? how much emphasis should be put on control of the diabetes or control of weight? how and when should oral hypoglycaemic drugs be used? is there a place for dietary fibre in the treatment of diabetes?

Opinion about carbohydrate restriction is becoming more liberal. The history of the dietary treatment of obesity has been reviewed by Leeds (1979): the earliest diets were low in energy and in carbohydrate. The importance of energy restriction in the obese diabetic is obvious, but there is no evidence that there is any advantage in restricting the contribution of carbohydrate to less than 45%, which is the average for a normal diet. Indeed Simpson et al (1979) recommend a diet in which 60% of the energy comes from carbohydrate, mostly of cereal or vegetable origin, but simple sugars are restricted. Wilson et al (1980) use a diet supplying 6 MJ (1400 kcal) of which 150 g is carbohydrate which supplies 42% of the energy. Genuth (1979) commends the supplemented fast, in which total energy intake is only 1.2 MJ (300 kcal) derived from 45 g egg albumin and 30 g sucrose daily. We do not know which diet will in the long run be associated with the fewest complications, but each can be shown to work well in the short term.

The emphasis to be put on control of the diabetes or of the obesity obviously depends on the relative severity of the two conditions. In the massively overweight diabetic it is reasonable to give priority to weight loss, since this is the only way in which the remaining insulin-secreting capacity can be conserved in the long run. It is tempting to permit such patients to excrete sugar in the urine, since this is another route of energy loss, but at present there is no evidence whether the accelerated weight loss which this would produce would be justified in view of the risk of uncontrolled diabetes and its long-term complications.

The usual advice is to use oral hypoglycaemic drugs when the obese diabetic 'cannot be controlled by diet alone' (Davidson et al 1979). This begs the question — how strict a diet, and how soon do you expect control? Genuth (1979) shows that patients who are taken off sulphonylurea drugs and put on a supplemented fast show a decline of blood sugar to normal levels over a period of several months, whereas previously untreated diabetics are normoglycaemic in 3 weeks. Patients tend to regard tablets as an easy alternative to dieting, and this view should be discouraged, but it seems reasonable to use oral agents (metformin rather than sulphonylureas) as an adjunct to diet to obtain better control of the diabetes when necessary. Certain forms of dietary fibre delay the absorption of sugar from the gut, and hence reduce the peak blood sugar levels after a meal (Leeds 1979). Whether this will prove useful in the long run remains to be seen.

DIETARY TREATMENT OF GRADE II OBESITY

Since the grade II obese person has about 15–45 kg (30–100 lb) of excess adipose tissue to lose, and since this adipose tissue represents a store of about 100,000–300,000 kcal (400–1200 MJ) the problem of treatment may be restated thus: 'How can this person be helped to maintain a negative energy balance of 1000 kcal/day for 100–300 days, or 500 kcal/day for 200–600 days?'. The theoretical basis of low-energy diets has been reviewed in the previous section: this section concerns the application of these principles. It is essential that the patient should understand the nature of the difficult task before him, and should be confident that the advice offered is effective and practicable. However, it is very unlikely that the grade II patient has had no advice before, so the first step is to find out what prejudices the patient holds, what lines of treatment have already been tried, and why these have failed. Armed with this knowledge it is more likely that advice can be given which will be seen to be relevant to the problems of that patient. If no proper history is taken, and advice is given which has already been tried and found ineffective, it is unlikely that the patient will retain any confidence in the therapist.

Assessment of previous therapeutic failures

The principles of investigation of the grade II patient are similar to those set out on page 63 for the grade III patient. However this assessment is even more important for the grade II patient who will need to be very strongly motivated to achieve substantial weight loss by voluntary restriction of energy intake. The rather crude therapeutic operations suggested in grade III have many disadvantages, but at least they make less demands on the willpower of the patient than a prolonged course of dieting.

First, measure the patient's weight and height, so the W/H^2 index can be calculated. Next ask the set of ten questions summarised in Table 5.6, from which the patient's motivation and expectations can be assessed. It is best to ask the questions and record the answers without comment, but if the question is evaded persist in asking it again.

1 'Why do you want to lose weight?' This may be rephrased 'What benefits do you think you would gain from losing weight?' or 'What things do you want to do, but are unable to do on account of your present weight?'

Try to obtain specific examples, rather than generalisations like 'I hate being fat' or 'I just feel generally uncomfortable'. Do not accept second-hand reasons: you want to know what reasons the patient has, not her doctor, friends or relatives.

2 'What weight do you think you should be?' Usually grade II patients will give an estimate near the upper part of the desirable range of weight-for-height. Those who have been to slimming clubs will promptly quote the mid-point of this range for their height, since this is a target weight they have been given by a club leader. If the weight given is unusually high or low ask why they have this target: low

Table 5.6   Questions to elicit motivation and expectations of grade II obese patients

Question	Information yielded
1 Reasons for losing weight? 2 Personal ideal weight?	Is expectation of benefit realistic?
3 Dieting at present? 4 Ever been heavier? 5 Longest diet? What result? 6 Expected rate of weight loss?	Were inappropriate methods used? Too rapid weight loss expected? Dieting given too low priority?
7 Family? Cooking? Shopping? 8 Any medication at present? 9 Expecting magic cure? 10 Nature of employment?	Are social circumstances such that dieting is impractical? Is mental/physical health such that weight loss would bring little benefit

estimates of ideal weight are usually related to weight at some halcyon period of youth, and high estimates to the weight they were immediately prior to the onset of their present disabilities.

3 'Are you on a diet at present?' The immediate answer to this question is worth recording: often it will be modified later. If the answer is 'yes' find out the nature of the diet, and for how long it has been observed. Is it simply 'being careful what I eat', or is there a defined calorie limit, or does it involve the conscientious ingestion of diet pills without any actual restriction on food intake?

4 'Is your present weight the maximum you have ever been?' If not what was the maximum, how long ago, and how was it reduced?

5 'Tell me about the longest time you have ever kept strictly to a reducing diet?' Record the nature of the diet, the duration, the weight loss achieved — from what weight to what weight, how long ago this effort was made, and why it was abandoned. This information may have been obtained already in answer to question 4.

6. 'If you keep strictly to a diet, how quickly do you think you should lose weight?' If the answer is 'I don't know', or 'Quite quickly at first, I should think, from my weight', try to get a quantitative answer by asking: 'After the first week or two, when you may lose weight quicker, do you think it is reasonable to expect on average to lose one, two, four pounds per week, or what?' Sometimes it is impossible to obtain any quantitative reply.

7 'Tell me about your family'. This deliberately vague question will elicit whatever aspect of the family the patient thinks is most relevant to the present problem: viz 'Both my parents are overweight' if genetic factors are considered important, 'I have two girls and a boy' if obesity is attributed to childbearing, or 'My eldest boy works night shifts and my husband is a milk-roundsman' if the social pattern of the family is such that meals are being prepared every hour of the night and day. If necessary elicit information on all these aspects, find out who does the shopping and cooking, and if other members of the family are inclined to be helpful in keeping the patient on a diet.

8 'Are you on any medication at present?' Note particularly anorectic drugs, diuretics, antidepressants, thyroid preparations, analgesics for arthritis, oral hypoglycaemic agents, steroids, contraceptives and anti-hypertensive drugs.

9 'Do you expect to lose weight without dieting?' Usually the reply is 'Of course not', but the question will sometimes reveal that the patient has pinned hopes on some magic cure. If this is so the fact must be unearthed, or the entire interview will be a failure, since (from the patient's viewpoint) the only topic of real interest was never mentioned.

10 'What work do you do?' The answer gives an indication of social circumstances and intellectual ability, and may reveal special circumstances (extensive travelling, shift work, business entertaining, employment in catering) which will affect the patients ability to adhere to a diet.

It takes about ten minutes to obtain answers to these ten questions from the averagely-articulate patient. This process does not represent a complete examination in itself, but I have found that there is a higher yield of useful information about grade II obese patients from these ten questions than from all the subsequent examination and laboratory investigations. It may be useful to draw attention to questions which are excluded from this list, although they occur in other screening Questionnaires, such as that of Levitz and Jordan (1973). The patient is not asked about her body image, or what she thinks other people think about her, although this information may be volunteered. She is not asked about the age of onset of her obesity or if at any period she was underweight. She is not asked about the ill-effects of previous dieting attempts, but again these may be volunteered. She is not asked about the psychological antecedents of her obesity, temptation foods, bingeing and feelings of guilt. There are three reasons for excluding questions of this sort. First, they take much longer than the ten rather factual questions listed above, because they are matters of opinion which provoke many supplementary questions from the patient about exactly what the question means and to what period it refers. Second, I do not think the answers, when they are obtained, are of any practical help in planning the appropriate line of treatment. Third, if the initial questions are directed to matters of social acceptability, age of onset of obesity, and psychological aspects of eating behaviour, the patient may reasonably infer that these are the factors which determine prognosis or which are likely to be changed by treatment. I believe that this inference is untrue and should not be fostered by questions which have no compensating advantage.

Routine medical history and examination

The questions directed towards previous attempts and failures to lose weight should be followed by the normal systematic enquiry about general health at present, previous health and investigations, smoking and drinking habits, and (where relevant) menstrual function. Physical examination of very obese patients is unsatisfactory, particularly when listening to the chest or palpating the abdomen, since the fat layer may obscure all but the grossest abnormality. However there is no excuse for not taking the blood pressure, observing the skin for evidence of thyroid or adrenal disease, noting operation scars, examining the hips and knees for evidence of osteoarthritis, and the ankles for oedema. The ocular fundi should be examined, and the urine tested for protein and sugar.

With this information it is possible to judge if the obese patient is simply an obese patient, or if there is significant pathology in addition to, and separate from, the obesity. Only a minority of obese patients will have a second pathology, but it is important to detect it. A thin patient with a bulging stomach due to an ovarian cyst will soon be diagnosed, but in an obese patient the diagnosis may not be considered. Obese patients may be weak from anaemia, leukaemia or renal failure and never be investigated because their symptoms were plausibly explained by obesity. Breathlessness and pain in weight-bearing joints are common features of severe obesity, but they may indicate other disease if the degree is disproportionate to the degree of obesity. The need to consider other pathology applies with all grades of obesity, but is perhaps most important in grade II, because in grade III it is likely that the diagnosis will be made anyway in the course of inpatient investigations, and in the lesser grades of obesity it is unlikely that the clues would be obscured by fatness.

Laboratory work-up
An algorithm for evaluating obese patients has been proposed by Bray et al (1976b). The flow chart indicates points at which laboratory tests should be used to screen for Cushing's syndrome, hypothyroidism, impaired glucose tolerance, hypoventilation, pituitary tumours and hyperlipidaemia. Obese patients may have all or any of these, and so may thin patients. Impaired glucose tolerance and hyperlipidaemia is certainly commoner among obese than among thin patients, but the management is in any case to treat the obesity, so whether the test is done or not the treatment is the same. Headaches, raised blood pressure and menstrual irregularities are common in obese patients: they tend to improve with weight loss, and skull X-ray and endocrine tests are usually within normal limits. If the diagnosis of Cushing's syndrome is never considered it will never be made, but it is extravagant to investigate every obese patient. It is worth doing laboratory tests if, on clinical grounds, there is reason to suspect the results will be abnormal, or alternatively when the patient is convinced that the root of the problem lies in (for example) hypothyroidism. It is easier and more effective to do the tests than to argue about it.

Deciding what advice to give
In the light of the information gleaned from the questions (Table 5.6) and medical and laboratory examinations a decision must be made: is it

worth while to attempt to treat this patient? Usually, with a grade II obese patient the answer will be Yes, since there are great benefits for most patients after weight loss. However there are some situations in which the effort is doomed to failure. If, in response to questions 1 and 2, it is obvious that the patients expectations of benefit are quite unrealistic, or their target weight is impossibly low, it is wise to correct these ideas before proceeding, otherwise the patient will in the end be disappointed. The patient is entitled to a well-informed and consistent estimate of benefits attainable.

If, in response to questions 3–6 it is clear that the patient has been conscientiously following some inappropriate method for achieving weight loss (sauna baths, electric treatment, exercise programmes, diuretics) this is a good sign, because with an effective method results should be better. However, if the patient has never made much effort, expects to lose weight without trying, or expects to lose weight at about 5 lb per week, these ideas must be modified before it is profitable to attempt treatment. Unless the patient is prepared to invest a reasonable amount of effort failure is certain.

Sometimes questions 7–10, or the medical or laboratory investigation, indicate that treatment is hardly worthwhile. In some patients the social situation is so stressful that they can barely cope, and have no emotional strength to spare for the added stress of dieting. Sometimes it is possible to improve the social situation by enlisting the help of other family members, or providing other forms of social support. In the case of severe mental or physical illhealth the benefit to be obtained from weight loss may be negligible. For example, in the Prader-Willi syndrome patients are often so mentally retarded that they are incapable of living independent lives, but require constant supervision. Much of their pleasure in life seems to come from eating. In such circumstances it is ineffective, and probably inhumane, to try to achieve much in the way of weight loss.

A problem may arise if the patient says that unless a weight loss of 5 lb per week is achieved something is wrong: such rates of weight loss have been achieved by others, and nothing less is acceptable. There is really no answer to this attitude but to say that if the patient wants to look elsewhere for such results he or she should do so. Most patients in this category return after a few months with a more realistic attitude to the rate of weight loss which can be expected.

Tailoring the diet to the patient: meal frequency
As a first guess, a diet supplying about 1000 kcal (4.2 MJ) daily for women, or 1500 kcal (6.3 MJ) for men, should produce weight loss of about the optimum rate. The principles on which such diets are based

are set out on pages 90–100. It is in the application of these principles to produce a diet which is acceptable and effective in a given patient that the professional skills of a dietitian are required. Any doctor who has access to trained dietetic help should use this facility. It is the dietitian's job to be skilled in taking a dietary history, to be familiar with the nutrient values of foods and how they are affected by different modes of cooking, and to be able to suggest alternative items of food to allow for individual preferences or religious or cultural factors. If no trained dietetic help is available, and the doctor wants to treat obese patients, the doctor must go to the trouble of acquiring these skills. It is absurd simply to hand over a diet sheet to an obese patient and to think that this constitutes adequate dietary advice.

One of the controversial aspects of reducing diets concerns the effect on weight loss of variations in meal frequency. It has been suggested that isoenergetic diets taken as a small number of large meals (gorging) cause more weight gain, or less weight loss, than when taken as a large number of small meals (nibbling), but the mechanism of this effect has not been explained (Fabry 1973). On theoretical grounds the reverse might be expected: if infrequent meals are taken the energy must be stored and then remobilised to meet metabolic demands, and this should require more metabolic work than a situation in which the energy supply is more or less continuous, so very little storage and mobilisation of energy stores is required. If the diets are identical in energy content, and the gorging mode is associated with the higher energy expenditure, then the gorging mode must be associated with the greater energy deficit and hence the greater rate of weight loss.

An investigation of the effect on weight loss and nitrogen balance of diets differing in meal frequency and protein concentration was reported by Garrow et al (1981). A total of 38 obese women were studied in a metabolic ward for 3 weeks. During the first week all the patients were given a diet supplying 800 kcal (3.4 MJ) with 13% of the energy as protein. This diet was served as three meals per day. During the second and third weeks, using a balanced cross-over design, the meal frequency was altered to one or five meals a day, or the protein concentration was altered to 10% or 15% of the total energy, or both changes were combined, so the isoenergetic diet was either one meal per day of 10% protein-energy, or five meals per day of 15% protein-energy.

The results of these dietary manipulations on weight loss are shown in Figure 5.11. The most rapid weight loss was achieved in those patients having one meal per day with 10% protein-energy, and as the meal frequency increased, and the protein concentration increased, there was a trend towards decreasing rate of weight loss. However it

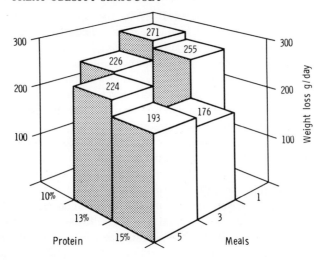

Fig. 5.11 Weight loss (g/day) among obese patients who were given a diet supplying 800 kcal (3.4 MJ) per day with either 10%, 13% or 15% of the energy as protein, served as either one, three or five meals per day (data of Garrow et al 1981). Infrequent meals of lower protein concentration are associated with more rapid weight loss

would be wrong to conclude that this type of diet is beneficial to the obese patient, for reasons which are shown in Figure 5.12. The nitrogen loss in the patients on the low-protein single-meal regimen was much greater than that with the more frequent meals of higher protein concentration. The extra weight loss can be entirely accounted for by extra loss of lean tissue, which is a disadvantage to the obese patient.

There are therefore two reasons for advising patients on a low-energy diet to have small frequent meals, rather than one large one. First, it appears that preservation of lean tissue is better with frequent meals, and second, hunger is less, for a given energy intake, if the meals are spread fairly evenly throughout the day. However there is no reliable information about the benefit to the patient of taking breakfast if he or she is not hungry in the early morning. It is normal teaching that omitting breakfast leads to greater hunger, and hence more overeating, in the remainder of the day, but there seems to be no published evidence for the truth of this dogma.

Apart from the meal pattern, the other respect in which it is possible to manipulate diets of equal energy content concerns the proportions of protein, carbohydrate and fat. The data in Figure 5.12 indicate that a fairly high protein concentration helps to preserve lean body mass, at least in the short term. The benefit of ketosis so far as protein-sparing

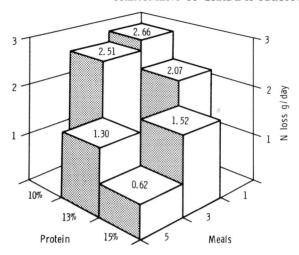

Fig. 5.12 Nitrogen loss (g/day) in the patients on the diets described in Figure 5.11. The more rapid weight loss associated with infrequent meals of lower protein concentration is entirely explained by more rapid loss of lean tissue in these patients. Frequent meals of higher protein concentration are more beneficial, because they are associated with greater sparing of lean tissue, and equally rapid fat loss (data of Garrow et al 1981)

is concerned is not established (see pp. 102–111), but may have some psychological value in patients who believe that 'cheating' on the diet will be unmasked if their urine is found to be free of ketones. This Big Brother approach is similar to that used by Kempner et al (1975) who use the presence of urinary sodium or chloride to detect deviation from their rice diet. It has been claimed that weight loss is greater on a relatively high-fat diet than on a diet of equal energy but with a high carbohydrate content (Rabast et al 1978) but this has not been confirmed in other careful studies (Yang & van Itallie 1976). Perhaps the most useful thing which can be said about removing carbohydrate, rather than other energy-yielding nutrients, from the diet is that thereby it is unlikely that the nutritive value of the diet will be greatly decreased (Stock & Yudkin 1970). The supplemented fasting programme of Vertes et al (1977b) provides 45 g protein and 30 g carbohydrate with vitamin and potassium supplements. This programme may well suit those patients who need to be removed from normal food if they are to achieve satisfactory weight loss.

ANORECTIC DRUG TREATMENT

Hunger is a cause of discomfort to patients on a low-energy diet. It is an effect of many drugs to impair appetite, but amphetamine and its related compounds are particularly potent in this respect. Of the 2,500,000 prescriptions written annually in the U.K. for anti-obesity drugs, at a cost to the National Health Service of £3.5m in 1975, most are for anorectic drugs, despite official advice that such medication 'is no substitute for willpower' (Munro 1979). This is true, but if anorectic drugs are even an effective aid to willpower this would be a good reason for prescribing them.

Psychopharmacology of anorectic drugs

The structural formulae for the most commonly used anorectic drugs are shown in Figure 5.13. The phenylethylamine skeleton is common to amphetamine, phentermine, diethylpropion and fenfluramine, and also to the neurotransmitters adrenalin and noradrenalin. Mazindol has an unrelated structure.

Amphetamine is a powerful stimulant of the central nervous system, and is liable to abuse, particularly among young people. In high doses it causes a syndrome similar to schizophrenia. For this reason prescription of amphetamine is controlled by the Misuse of Drugs Act, 1971, in the U.K., and by an agreement among practitioners to avoid its use in the treatment of obesity (Munro 1979). In the U.S. it is on Schedule II of the Drug Enforcement Administration (Sullivan and Comai 1978).

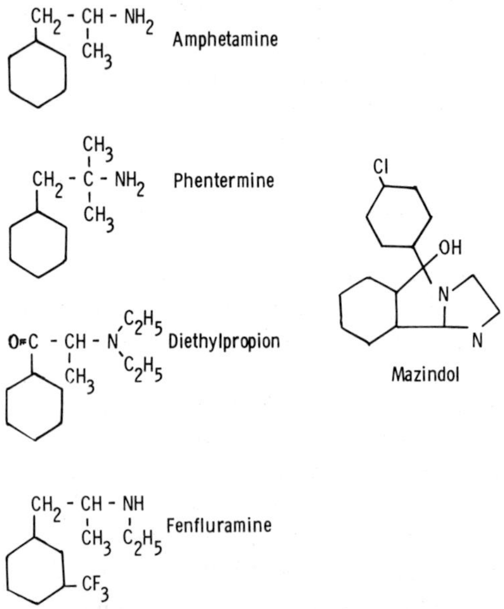

Fig. 5.13 The structural formulae of commonly-used anorectic drugs.

Modification of the side chain of amphetamine yields the compounds phentermine and diethylpropion, which retain much of the anorectic potency of amphetamine, but with greatly reduced potential for abuse: both these drugs are on Schedule IV of the Drug Enforcement Administration (Sullivan and Comai 1978). Although these drugs are less powerfully stimulant than amphetamine their side effects are similar in type: sleeplessness, palpitations, dry mouth, nervousness and irritability. However fenfluramine, which is also on Schedule IV of the Drug Enforcement Administration, is not at all stimulant. The insertion of a fluoryl group at the 3 position in the phenol ring alters the mode of action and clinical effects of the drug. The side effects of fenfluramine are drowsiness, diarrhoea, and depression which is most likely to occur on sudden withdrawal of the drug (Steel and Briggs 1972).

Mazindol is a novel compound, which is rated by the Drug Enforcement Administration in Schedule III, between amphetamine and the other compounds in potential for abuse. Many side effects have been reported (Munro 1979) but there is less experience of long-term administration of mazindol than with the other compounds.

The mode of action of anorectic drugs has been extensively reviewed (Garattini and Samanin 1976, Blundell and Burridge 1979). Amphetamine and fenfluramine are the two compounds which have been most thoroughly studied. In general amphetamine suppresses hunger, so that feeding is postponed, while fenfluramine enhances satiety, so the meal size is reduced. However the mode of action which produces these effects is still not clear, since the action of amphetamine changes with dose level (Blundell and Burridge 1979). While amphetamine, phentermine, diethylpropion and mazindol act on catecholamine neurotransmitters in the brain, fenfluramine interacts with brain serotonin (Garattini and Samanin 1976).

Results of treatment with anorectic drugs

There is no doubt that well-controlled double-blind trials have shown significantly greater weight loss in obese patients who were given anorectic drugs than in control subjects who were given placebo medication. A survey by the U.S. Food and Drug Administration showed that 44% of patients on drugs achieved a weight loss of 1 lb (0.45 kg) per week, compared with only 26% of patients on placebo: the addition of an anorectic drug resulted in an extra weight loss of 0.23 kg per week (Sullivan and Comai 1978). No significant differences were observed in the weight loss achieved by any of the drugs examined.

Unfortunately these results apply to trials which are rarely more than 12 weeks in duration, and the weight loss achieved is typically about 6 kg with the active drug, and about 3 kg with placebo. The combination of a diet sheet and an anorectic drug is not going to solve the problem of the grade II obese patient, who has at least 15 kg to lose.

Drug trials of longer duration are disheartening for two reasons: first, the rate of weight loss steadily decreases, and second, it is hard work to prevent excessive numbers of patients from dropping out and thereby invalidating the trial. One of the best trials was that of Steel et al (1973) who studied a series of 105 patients for 36 weeks with only 23% dropout, which is a tribute to the thoroughness with which the patients were supervised. Any patient who did not keep an appointment was immediately sent a letter, and if this elicited no response the physician conducting the trial visited the patient at home. The schedules of medication which were tested were continuous fenfluramine, fenfluramine and placebo on alternate months, alternate fenfluramine and phentermine, phentermine and placebo on alternate months, and finally fenfluramine and phentermine alternating with placebo in the intervening months. The greatest weight loss (12 kg) was achieved in the continuous fenfluramine and the alternate phentermine and placebo regimens. Intermittent fenfluramine is unsatisfactory, since it causes too severe side effects. Although these results are probably the best reported for an anorectic drug trial (Wing and Jeffrey 1979) it should be noted that the patients were advised to keep to a diet supplying 1000 kcal (4.2 MJ) daily, and were closely supervised. Furthermore, this trial shows well the decreasing rate of weight loss: in the first 6 months the patients on continuous fenfluramine lost on average 10.8 kg, and in the last 3 months they lost only another 2.3 kg. In the case of the group treated with intermittent phentermine weight loss was 10.9 kg in the first six months and 1.1 kg in the last 3 months.

The problem of maintaining the weight loss achieved with the help of anorectic drugs has been discussed by Munro (1979). There is no evidence that a course of drugs 'retrains eating habits' in any permanent way: indeed the evidence is that when the drug is stopped weight is quite rapidly regained. Munro argues that there is a good case for continuing the administration of the drug indefinitely, if this is what is required to maintain the weight loss. The disadvantages of this plan are that it is expensive, and there is no good evidence that the weight loss would be maintained, or that the patients would continue to take the drug indefinitely.

It might be supposed that anorectic drugs would be a very popular method of weight loss so far as obese patients were concerned, since it involves less of a strain on the willpower of the patient. However this was not the conclusion reached by Ashwell (1973) from the response of

1,362 patients to a questionnaire about their views on doctors' treatment of obesity: most patients who had experience of both methods said that as a means of attaining permanent weight loss they preferred diet alone to diet assisted by drugs.

It has been suggested that the weight loss induced by drugs such as fenfluramine may not be attributable entirely to an anorectic effect, since these drugs have been shown to have effects on glucose and lipid metabolism in man (Turner 1978). It has been pointed out on page 18 that ultimately the gain or loss of fat must depend on a change in energy balance, whatever may happen in intermediary metabolism. Thus if a drug causes fat loss by some means other than by reducing energy intake it must increase energy expenditure. Such studies as have been done on fenfluramine given to patients on a constant energy intake have failed to show any such effect (Garrow et al 1972, Wales 1980).

Combined anorectic drugs and behaviour modification

Behaviour modification (See pp. 140-5) seeks to give patients better control over food intake, with a view to achieving lasting weight loss. It is therefore logical to try a combination of anorectic drugs and behaviour modification, the former to help to achieve weight loss, and the latter to help to maintain it. A very interesting study by Stunkard et al (1980) suggests that the two modes of treatment do not combine in this beneficial way. They studied 134 men and women recruited by advertisement, many of whom were hypertensive. The subjects paid a deposit of $25 to discourage drop-out. Behaviour modification was along the lines described on pages 140-141, and drug therapy was fenfluramine continuously up to a dose of 120 mg per day: some patients had only behaviour modification, some only fenfluramine, and some had both combined. The weight loss in six months by the behaviour modification group was 10.9 ± 1.0 kg (Mean $\pm$ S.E.M.) and in the drug and combined group it was 14.4 ± 1.1 kg and 15.3 ± 1.2 kg respectively. These excellent weight losses may be attributed to the high dose of fenfluramine (Steel et al 1973 used only 60 mg per day) and to the close supervision of the patients who met in groups for 1½ hours each week under the guidance of trained psychologists and a dietitian who advised them on a diet supplying 1000-1200 kcal (4.2-5.0 MJ) per day.

Although the groups who had fenfluramine lost more weight than those treated purely by behaviour modification during the six months of treatment, the situation was reversed after another twelve months of follow-up. The behaviour therapy patients regained only 1.9 ± 1.0 kg, while the drug group regained 8.2 ± 1.2 kg and the combined treatment group 10.7 ± 1.2 kg. The authors comment that this result favours behaviour therapy over drug therapy, and certainly it suggests that the addition of an anorectic drug to behaviour modification destroys the beneficial long-term learning effect of behaviour modification. It is noticeable that in the two months after the cessation of treatment the behaviour therapy group continued to lose another 2 kg, while both the groups treated with drugs gained 2 kg, thereby closing the 4 kg gap between them at the end of the treatment period.

The potency of placebo medication

A remarkable feature of the drug treatment of obesity is the effectiveness of pharmacologically inert substances when administered in impressive circumstances. Wing and Jeffery (1979) note that the weight loss of 6.5 kg in a group of subjects who were receiving placebo injections six times a week (as a control for a group receiving human chorionic gonadotrophin) is superior to the weight loss achieved by most 'active' medications. Munro et al (1968) showed that the weight loss in a group of patients who were given alternate phentermine and dummy tablets monthly for 9 months was actually slightly greater than that achieved by patients taking continuous phentermine, although their data clearly show that weight loss during the placebo months of this alternating regimen was less than during the months of active medication. They suggest that the intermittent therapy delayed the onset of tolerance to the drug. However Stunkard (1978) disputes the idea that a decreasing rate of weight loss with prolonged administration of an anorectic drug is valid evidence of tolerance. If it were true that the drug ceased to have any effect after, say, 9 months administration, then stopping the drug at that stage should have no effect either. In fact stopping anorectic treatment is promptly followed by weight increase, which is evidence that the drug was doing something, if not still causing weight loss. In the light of this observation it is all the more intriguing that placebo medication should achieve weight loss.

A plausible explanation is that placebo medication has an important effect on the morale of the dieting patient. Any factor which helps the patient to believe that this time the effort to lose weight will be successful, however many previous attempts have failed, may assist the resolve to diet and hence lose weight. This view is supported by the observation of Atkinson et al (1977) who reported no difference in weight loss achieved with anorectic drugs or placebo, but a significant difference according to the therapist administering treatment. The amount a patient eats depends on at least two factors: the actual level of hunger, which may be influenced by drug action, and the motivation of the patient to ovecome this hunger, which is influenced greatly by the charisma of the therapy or the therapist. Any treatment, however absurd, will have some measure of success if it has an element of magic about it.

Another interesting effect of drug therapy is that it tends to decrease drop-out from outpatient clinics. Figure 5.14 shows the percentage of patients still attending one, three and six months after first attending an obesity clinic as National Health Service patients. The patients were randomly assigned to one of three treatment groups: a control group was given standard dietary advice without any medication, another group was given tablets each month, some of which were active and some placebo in a double-blind fashion, and a third group was offered behaviour therapy, which involved more frequent attendance at hospital. Among both men and women the attendance of those given tablets fell off less rapidly than among the control group.

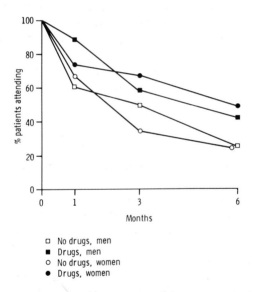

Fig. 5.14 The effect of prescription of a drug or placebo (in a double-blind trial) on drop-out rate among obese patients at a hospital obesity clinic

The patients who were given tablets had either two months of active and one of placebo in each 3-month cycle, or else one month active and two months placebo. The attendance record was similar in the two groups: 3.3 ± 1.7 months for those with two out of three months on active tablets, and 3.4 ± 2.2 months for those with one out of three months on active tablets. Count of returned tablets showed no difference in the number of tablets taken per month: 22 ± 10 tablets per 4 weeks for active, and 19 ± 9 per 4 weeks for placebo tablets. Although there was a greater weight loss during the months on active tablets than months on placebo (2.1 ± 2.7 kg vs 0.9 ± 2.4 kg, P<0.05) the overall weight loss was not significantly different between those on the frequent, or infrequent, active tablet schedule. Out of a series of 9 men and 39 women who entered this trial only four continued to take the medication and return the bottles for tablet counts for 9 months. Figure 5.15 shows the weight loss, type of tablet provided, and number of tablets taken per four-week period by these four individuals.

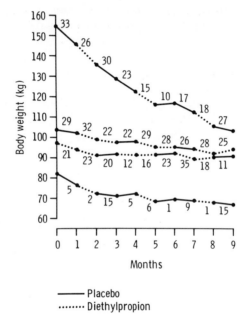

Fig. 5.15 Weight loss, and number of tablets per month, in 4 patients who took 75 mg slow-release diethylpropion (broken line) or placebo (solid line) for 9 months in a double-blind trial

These results suggest that for a minority of patients anorectic drugs are helpful, but that they are probably best used intermittently over a long period. There is little to be said for short sharp courses of anorectic drugs. It is important to note that fenfluramine is not suitable for this intermittent use, since depression is an important complication on stopping this drug (Steel and Briggs 1972).

THERMOGENIC DRUGS AND ENERGY-LOSING TREATMENTS

The objective of treatment in obesity is to create a negative energy balance, so the patient burns excess fat stores. The alternative to reducing energy intake is to increase energy losses. This may be achieved either by increasing the metabolic rate with exercise or thermogenic drugs, or else by impairing the absorption of food from the gut so more energy is lost in faeces. The effect of exercise on energy balance is considered in Chapter 6, but the use of drugs to increase energy losses will be considered here.

There are several drugs which cause transient increase in metabolic rate, but the group which are clinically most effective are the thyroid hormones. If thyroxine is given in excess of physiological requirement the metabolic rate is increased to a variable extent, since conversion of thyroxine to the active triiodothyronine, or the inactive reverse-triiodothyronine, provides a method of regulation of the biological effect. If triiodothyronine is given there is no scope for this type of regulation. At the dosage of thyroid hormone required to achieve significant weight loss toxic symptoms are common, and the extra weight lost is mostly lean tissue rather than fat (Bray et al 1971). Even if this loss of lean tissue is prevented there is danger of damage to heart muscle with thyroid intoxication (Sullivan and Comai 1978).

An alternative use of thyroid hormone is to prevent the decrease in metabolic rate which is associated with low-energy diets (Garrow 1974, Moore et al 1980). Even at the relatively modest dosage of 120 μg per day of triiodothyronine there is a marked increase in nitrogen loss from the body (Warwick and Garrow 1981). The long-term results of treatment of obesity with thyroxine are no better than those of diet alone (Sullivan and Comai 1978), and the administration of thyroxine to euthyroid patients merely makes difficulties in the interpretation of subsequent thyroid function tests. True hypothyroidism occurs no more frequently in obese people than among lean people (Strata et al 1978).

Since it is suggested that the site of dietary thermogenesis is brown fat (Rothwell and Stock 1979), and that the metabolic activity of this tissue is modulated by catecholamines, there is renewed interest in the thermogenic potential of sympathomimetic drugs. Evans and Miller (1977) showed in acute experiments that ephidrene in a dose of 44 mg orally caused an increase in resting metabolic rate of about 10%, and also enhanced the thermogenic response to a meal. So far there is no evidence that this effect would be of practical use in treating obesity.

The results of controlled trials suggest that the action of human chorionic gonadotrophin in the treatment of obesity is not different from that of a placebo (Sullivan and Comai 1978), but since it is administered frequently, and by injection, this placebo effect may be strong (Wing and Jeffery 1979).

At present, therefore, there is little evidence that drugs which increase metabolic rate are clinically useful in treating obesity, and they all must carry some risk. One of the disadvantages of obesity is that the patient's exercise tolerance is decreased, because even at rest there is less cardiac reserve than in a person of normal weight. Any drug which further increases resting metabolism in an obese patient must further decrease this reserve.

It is theoretically possible that a drug may be found which will inhibit the absorption of nutrients from the gut. Such compounds have already been tested in animals (Sullivan and Comai 1978). These compounds will cause weight loss, but the dietary energy which is made unavailable to the patient becomes available to colonic bacteria, so it is foreseeable that extensive colonic fermentation and gas production will be an inevitable side effect of any such form of drug therapy.

BEHAVIOUR MODIFICATION

The paper by Stuart (1967) on 'The behavioral control of overeating' seemed to mark the beginning of a new era in the treatment of obesity. There have been many new treatments for obesity, but this one reported a series of 8 patients who lost 17 ± 4 kg over a period of 12 months — results which had not previously been attained except by surgical or inpatient treatments. The essential features of Stuart's programme were that the patient had to keep detailed records of the time, nature, quantity and circumstance of all food and drink intake, and a record of weight before breakfast, after breakfast, after lunch and before bedtime. At first the patient had three 30-minute sessions with the therapist each week, at which she learned to make the process of eating progressively more formalised and less spontaneous: she had to stop for 5 minutes in the middle of each meal, only one food portion at a time was to be prepared, eating was made a pure experience and not an incidental activity while listening to the radio. As therapy went on sessions were more widely spaced, so the 8 patients had from 16 to 41 sessions in all.

It was obvious that this intensity of treatment was impractical except for those obese patients who were willing and able to retain the full-time services of a therapist: 'The therapist is available by telephone at all times, in order to guard against any failure by the patient which might adversely affect his expectation of success' (Stuart 1967). However controlled trials of behavioural techniques against traditional group psychotherapy, with equal exposure to the therapist in both cases, showed better weight loss in the behaviour therapy group (Penick et al 1971), but never the spectacular losses reported in Stuart's original paper.

Many attempts were made to modify the behavioural programme to make it less extravagant in therapist time. One obvious step was to treat patients in groups, rather than individually (Blake 1976). The main features which behavioural programmes have in common are an agreement to keep records of food intake and weight change, an attempt to restrict cues which cause eating and to eat more slowly, and various systems for rewarding these changes in behaviour. However it requires considerable dedication on the part of the patient to carry out these procedures conscientiously, so attempts have been made to increase the commitment of patients by requiring a monetary deposit, which is returnable gradually if the programme is followed. There is no doubt that the stronger the monetary contracts the better the results obtained (Jeffery et al 1978) but it is not clear if the deposits increase motivation, or merely select those patients who are already highly motivated. Obviously a person who is willing to stake a substantial sum of money at the beginning of treatment is serious at that stage, while a person who was less wholehearted in his desire to lose weight would not enter the programme. Involvement of the patient's spouse in the treatment process may help (Wilson and Brownell 1978) or it may have no significant effect (O'Neil et al 1979).

Attempts have been made to find out which of the components in the behavioural programme are the most effective in producing weight loss, but no clear answer emerges. For example Loro et al (1979) assigned 110 moderately obese subjects to one of three treatment groups: one concentrated on eating behaviour — decreasing portion sizes and eating slowly; another group concentrated on removing food cues; the third kept a weight graph and were encouraged to develop their own strategies to achieve target weight. Monetary deposits kept the dropout rate below 10% in all groups. The authors present a statistical analysis showing that the third group did best, but inspection of their data shows that this group lost weight more rapidly in the pre-treatment baseline week than at any other stage in the study.

Although no subsequent publications on behaviour modification have been able to match the spectacular weight losses of Stuart (1967) interest has centred on the ability of behavioural methods to produce sustained weight loss. 'The shortcoming of behavioral programs has been the small losses achieved; the record of maintenance is, by contrast, impressive' (Wooley et al 1980), and 'Despite modest weight losses, behavior modification approaches continue to be of interest because of their good record in maintaining weight loss during follow-up' (Wing and Jeffery 1979). However, even this claim requires careful study. If the weight loss achieved in treatment is trivial, then it is of trivial importance whether or not it is maintained. Götestam (1979) reports a 3-year follow-up of 11 patients treated with behaviour modification, who lost on average 9.4 kg during a 16 week treatment programme. One year later they had regained 4.8 kg on average, but as a group they were still significantly below their pre-treatment weight. At the 3 year follow-up they were on average only 2.1 kg below pre-treatment weight, and this was not significantly different from zero weight loss. Stunkard and Penick (1979) have reviewed the long-term weight loss achieved in ten publications based on behavioural techniques, including a five-year follow-up of one of their own series. At one year their series of patients treated by behavioural and traditional methods had lost, on average, 12.6 and 12.1 kg respectively, but at 5 years this had reduced to a mean loss of 5.3 and 5.5 kg respectively. In only 4 of the 10 studies reviewed by Stunkard and Penick (1979) was the median weight loss greater than 6.4 kg, and they conclude that 'clinically important weight losses achieved by behavioural treatments are not well maintained'. In those studies in which little weight was lost during the treatment period the results on follow-up are equally discouraging.

All this suggests that behavioural modification is not in itself a satisfactory treatment for grade II obesity, but it is important to look for clues to the success which has been achieved by this technique. For those who enjoy studying their own psychology and personality, and who have the leisure to keep the required records, behaviour modification is much more attractive than merely following dietary advice. However, as Weisenberg and Frey (1974) point out, it is not to be expected that less sophisticated patients will be willing or able to follow the programme. The advice that the patient should interrupt his meal for a predetermined time, initially 2 or 3 minutes which is gradually increased to 5 minutes, and 'put down his utensils and merely sit in his place at the table for a specified period of time' (Stuart 1967) assumes that the patient's family will tolerate this behaviour: it is not very practical for the average housewife who is feeding her family who may well believe that they have more urgent things to do than watch this demonstration of self-control at every meal.

A major contribution of the behaviourist school has been the recognition that the treatment of obesity does involve a change in eating behaviour, and that such change is difficult to achieve, and requires constant reinforcement to sustain. The old-fashioned and rather petulant view of the didactic nutritionist school, that if patients could not keep to the diet for even one month 'they had better be happy and fat' (Gray and Kallenbach 1939) is naive: obese patients are not happy, or they would not present as patients. However it is one thing to recognise the need for help with changing behaviour, but another to be able to provide that help. Ideally there should be constant reward for controlled behaviour, and initially this can be provided by the feeling of accomplishment as the behavioural steps are mastered, the praise of the therapist, and the evident weight loss. However this source of reinforcement fades with time: there are no new steps to master, weight loss gets slower, and the therapist may well have transferred some of his enthusiasm to other new patients who are making better progress, and who are themselves more enthusiastic.

Motivation may be sustained by 'contingency contracting', which is the psychologists' term for blackmail-by-consent. The patient agrees to some sanction which the therapist can impose if the patient defaults from the programme, but it is difficult to devise a sanction sufficiently severe to obtain compliance without getting into a situation in which the cure is worse than the disease. In a captive population these sanctions are effective: Bernard (1968) caused a scizophrenic patient to lose 46.3 kg in 6 months by imposing a system in which telephone calls, admission to dances, etc. had to be paid for with tokens, and the tokens had to be earned by weight loss. Policemen who were ordered to lose weight did so, since the alternative was loss of leave, money and promotion prospects (Scrignar 1980). There is an ethical problem in treating obese patients who are free agents, but who are seeking to have their behaviour changed: this is discussed in section 2.d and Chapter 10, since it applies also to the justification for surgical procedures or long inpatient treatments. Concerning contingency contracting in behaviour therapy it can be said that it helps while the contract is in force, but that when the contract expires weight is regained (Abramson 1977).

One source of reward which is, in principle, constantly renewable is the continued interest and support of the therapist. Lindstrom et al (1976) found that telephone contact was almost as good as in-person contact, but in their series weight loss was small (3 kg). Ashby and Wilson (1977) tried to sustain the effect of a behavioural programme with 'booster sessions', but with little effect in maintaining weight loss.

Perhaps the most serious criticism of behaviour modification is the total disregard, or even ignorance, which many of its practioners show for the principles of energy balance. It is assumed that obese patients are obese because they lack 'normal' control over eating: obesity is an 'eating disorder' (Stunkard 1972). It was no part of Stuart's plan to enquire what his patients ate, or to advise them what to eat: 'At the request of one patient the services of a dietitian was contracted for an hour ... This service is of help, but not essential' (Stuart 1967). It is assumed that the objective is to wrest the patient away from 'her pathological eating patterns' (Strain and Strain 1979), and then all will be well. There are three flaws in this argument.

First, most (but not all) obese patients have eating patterns which are indistinguishable from those of normal-weight people (Garrow 1978a, Durrant 1980). Many investigators have studied the eating pattern of lean and obese people, and while some have found differences others have not. It is certain that if a videotape was made of every particle of food consumed by an assorted group of subjects it would be impossible for an independent observer to deduce from the eating pattern if the subject to which it referred was fat or thin. It is true that some obese patients, when their resolution to diet collapses, indulge in spectacular eating binges. We do not know if lean people would behave similarly after a similar period of deprivation, since a controlled trial has not been done. From the experience in Germany after the war (Widdowson 1951) and with experimental undernutrition of lean volunteers (Keys et al 1950), it seems that the tendency to overeat on a massive scale after a period of food deprivation is not a characteristic limited to obese people.

The second flaw in the behavioural argument is that critical analysis of those studies in which both weight change and behaviour change have been recorded shows no convincing association between these two variables (Brownell and Stunkard 1978a). This is not surprising: a change in eating behaviour is necessary, but not necessarily sufficient, to cause weight loss. Weight loss depends on the extent to which the energy supplied by the diet fails to meet energy requirements (Chapter 3). It is obviously possible to eat slowly, in a formalised way, pausing between courses, without distracting influences like the radio, and to record meticulously what, where and how you have eaten, but still to take in enough food to meet your energy requirements. In such circumstances behaviour modification will not achieve weight loss. It is significant that in trials in which comparisons have been made between emphasising behavioural change or emphasising achieving weight loss (Mahoney 1974, Hall et al 1977, Loro et al 1979) it is the group oriented to weight loss which gets the better results.

Third, it must be acknowledged that what is being asked of the obese patient is not simply to acquire 'normal' control of eating. It is difficult to define what normal regulation of energy intake means, for reasons already given on pp. 35–38, but a consequence of normal regulation is a roughly constant body weight, achieved by matching intake to requirements. This is not enough for the patient with grade II obesity: here the target is to eat less than requirements to the tune of 100,000–300,000 kcal (400–1200 MJ), since that is the burden of excess fat which must be burned. Therefore it is misleading in theory, and ineffective in practice, to imply that behaviour modification will cure obesity by changing the 'pathological' eating patterns of the obese person into 'normal' ones. There is no magic about behavioural methods other than their effect on energy intake: Ritt et al (1979) analysed the diet records of 15 of the most successful members of a behaviour therapy group and concluded that their intake had decreased from 2067 kcal (8.64 MJ) to 1219 kcal (5.09 MJ) over a period of 15 weeks. If we assume that they were in energy balance on 2067 kcal, then on the reduced intake they would accumulate a deficit of $(2067-1219) \times 7 \times 15 = 89,000$ kcal in 15 weeks, and we might expect a weight loss of $89,000/7000 = 12.72$ kg. This agrees quite well with the reported loss of 14.2 kg in this group of subjects.

In those studies in which behaviour therapy has been compared with anorectic drugs the results have usually been better with behaviour therapy. Öst and Götestam (1976) achieved a weight loss of 9.4 kg in a 16 week behavioural group, with 4.6 kg mean loss remaining after one year. In a group treated with anorectic drugs the losses were 5.7 kg at 16 weeks and only 0.8 kg at one year. The trial of Dahms et al (1978) was marred by a high drop-out rate: of 120 patients enrolled only 33 completed a 14 week course. However the results show a slightly more favourable weight loss in the group treated with behaviour therapy than in those treated with either mazindol or diethylpropion.

HYPNOSIS AND OTHER FORMS OF PSYCHOTHERAPY

The term 'psychotherapy' can be interpreted very widely indeed. In his book *The art of psychotherapy* Storr (1979) defines it as 'the art of alleviating personal difficulties through the agency of words and a personal, professional relationship'. In this sense any doctor who talks sensibly and constructively to his patient, and who listens sympathetically to what the patient has to say, is engaged in psychotherapy. So wide a definition makes it difficult to say exactly where the expertise of the professional psychotherapist lies:

'Psychotherapy has been described as a treatment of unknown nature applied to conditions of uncertain origin with an unproved outcome, for which many years of rigorous training was required'. (Pond 1979).

There is certainly a need for psychotherapy for the people whose suffering arises not from obesity in itself, but from the 'stigma of overweight in everyday life' (Allon 1975). This is discussed further in Chapter 7: the present section is concerned with lines of treatment which will help obese people to lose weight.

Hypnosis is a form of treatment for obesity which is advertised to the public and it may well be helpful, but there are remarkably few reports which give detailed results and follow-up, and apparently no published trial in which hypnosis has been compared with some other mode of treatment (Mott and Roberts 1979). One of the early reports is by Winkelstein (1959) who treated 42 women, aged 16–52 years, who were found to be easily hypnotised and who were 10 to 60 lb above ideal weight. He implanted post-hypnotic suggestions that they would eat less and desire less food. At first these post-hypnotic suggestions lasted less than 24 hours, but with repeated reinforcement they became longer-lasting, and could be maintained by weekly hypnotism sessions. Over a 14 week period everyone in the group lost weight: on average the weight loss was about 20 lb (9 kg) and this loss was maintained (but did not increase) for another 14 weeks after the end of the treatment period. These results are quite encouraging, but it is not clear what proportion of all obese patients would be in the 'easily hypnotisable' category chosen by Winkelstein.

Stanton (1975) reports a follow up to 2 years on 10 out of 'many successful patients': they fell in weight from 71.5 to 65.2 kg in a period of 4 weeks of hypnotic treatment, and 6 months and 2 years later they were at 61.6 kg. Stanton (1976) suggested that fee-paying clients lost more weight than those who were treated free (9.05 kg vs 5.05 kg in 4 weeks). These rates of weight loss seem suspiciously high, and it is a pity that the reports are not based on a wider sample of Stanton's experience.

Probably the most helpful paper is by Aja (1977) which gives a verbatim account of the therapy procedure. It consisted of a 3 session treatment completed in a week, with instructions for ancillary self-hypnosis thereafter. Of the 40 patients in the trial (there is no mention of any drop-out) the starting weight was 104 kg, and the average loss at 3 months was 5.7 kg and at six months the average loss compared with pretreatment weight was 4.3 kg. The suggestion implanted under hypnosis was that clients should reject 'fattening and unnecessary' foods, and that they should adopt the formalised eating behaviours suggested by Stuart (1967).

Several workers used hypnosis as a means for applying aversion therapy. Tilker and Meyer (1972) provide an anecdotal account of one patient who was made to feel nausea when confronted with 'fattening' food, and Miller (1954) said he treated 50 patients who were trained to be nauseated by 'poisonous, ugly, fat-producing food' and in whom 'weight loss varied from 1-5 kg per week', but there is no analysis of the overall effect of this treatment. Meyer and Crisp (1964) and Foreyt and Kennedy (1971) also used aversion therapy to treat obese patients, but without hypnosis: patients were trained to reject 'temptation foods' by having them associated with punishment by electric shocks, or by noxious smells, respectively. In neither paper was a significant and sustained weight loss obtained. Rand and Stunkard (1978) observed that of 84 obese patients undergoing psychoanalysis 47% had lost more than 9 kg, and 19% had lost more than 18 kg, in a treatment period of 42 months.

It seems that the potentialities of hypnosis as a treatment for obesity have not been systematically investigated. It may be that the behaviour required of an obese person on a reducing diet is too sophisticated to be implanted by a few hypnotic commands, but the reports reviewed above take a very naive view of dietary treatment: what exactly is the patient to regard as a 'fattening food'? At least this literature reveals what must be the Most Easily Satisfied Therapist: this title must go to Ringrose (1979) who reports that 'Hypnotherapy ... has proved to be an excellent aid in curbing obesity'. He bases this conclusion on a personal series of 159 subjects. After 2 weeks attrition left him with only 63, and after 3 weeks there were 13, of whom 1 had lost 3–4% of initial weight, 11 had lost 1–2%, and one had lost nothing.

6

Management of grade I obesity

THE PUBLIC HEALTH SIGNIFICANCE
OF MODERATE OBESITY

Between one quarter and one third of the adult population of the
United Kingdom (James 1976), and of the United States (Bray 1979)
is moderately overweight: by the definition used in this book grade I
obesity applies to people whose W/H^2 lies between 25 and 30. There is
little evidence that this degree of moderate obesity carries any
significant health hazard for people over the age of 50 years, but it is
worth taking some trouble about moderate obesity in young people for
three reasons. First, the data of Blair and Haines (1966) show a
significant increase in mortality among young people who were only
moderately overweight (see Table 2.1, page 13). Second, it is
probable that a given investment of effort directed towards checking
obesity at stage I will show a better return than the same amount of
effort directed towards treating obesity which has reached stage II
or III. Third, although the mortality associated with grade I obesity is
not marked, there are social disadvantages attached to moderate
overweight (Allon 1975, DeJong 1980, Wooley et al 1980). In a
survey of slimmers by the Consumers' Association in the U.K. 58% of
women, but only 19% of men, wanted to lose weight for the sake of
looks or to have more choice of clothes: more men than women wanted
to lose weight for health reasons. Those who wanted to lose weight to
improve their appearance were less overweight than those who were
slimming for health reasons (Rudinger 1978).

In view of the vast number of people who are moderately obese it is
impractical to offer individual investigation and treatment, as
suggested for the more severe, and less common, degrees of obesity.
Fortunately this is not necessary. Well-designed community health
programmes, based on radio, television and printed media, make a
measurable impact on the weight and dietary habits of a community
(Farquhar 1978). A report by Stamler et al (1980) shows that the
Chicago Coronary Prevention Program, started in 1958, has produced

significant decrease in weight as well as in other coronary risk factors such as hypertension, hypercholesterolaemia, cigarette smoking and physical inactivity, and these changes persist for 9 years after entry into the programme. Change in weight and change in blood pressure were significantly correlated.

The effectiveness of health programmes may be enhanced or decreased according to the attitude of other health professionals with whom the public comes in contact. If a doctor dismisses as nonsense the advice that a moderately overweight person should try to reduce, it is unlikely that the health propaganda will have much effect. However if a doctor provides moral support for the idea of weight reduction it is much more likely that the patient will make the necessary effort.

THE ROLE OF THE GENERAL PRACTITIONER IN MANAGING GRADE I OBESITY

Bolden (1975), in an article entitled 'Against the active treatment of obesity in general practice' concludes:

'Because the present methods of treatment are so inefficient, I propose that weight reduction programmes for the average patient in general practice are worthless. We, as a profession, are hidebound by our traditions. It is time we took a long hard look at fruitless areas of therapeutic activity and asked ourselves if our efforts might not be better directed elsewhere'.

We do not know what proportion of general practitioners agree with this view. Where, for example, would their efforts be better directed? If it is beneath the dignity of general practitioners to treat obesity, whose job should it be?

Some light on these questions is given by the survey of Ashwell (1973) who analysed the replies of 2,333 people to a questionnaire from the Consumers' Association about methods of slimming. Most of those replying were grade I obese. Only 1362 of the respondents, 1117 women and 245 men, had received advice from a doctor about weight loss. About half the women, and a quarter of the men, had specifically sought advice about their weight: the remainder had gone about some other problem and been advised to lose weight. It appears, therefore, that in more than half the cases it was the doctor who suggested weight loss. Furthermore, since only 7% of the patients were advised to join a slimming group, 1% were referred to a hospital obesity clinic and 9% were advised not to worry about their weight, it follows that the general practitioner himself offered treatment to the remaining 83% of patients. Since we do not know the actual excess weight, and other medical problems of these patients, it is impossible to say if this was a reasonable arrangement.

It is certainly not reasonable that (if the replies are to be believed) only 28% of patients were asked to go back at regular intervals to be weighed. This is hard to understand. It takes very little time to weigh a patient. The measurement can easily be done by a trained assistant. The doctor who does not keep an accurate record of the patient's weight change every 2–4 weeks cannot claim to be treating obesity seriously, and has no right to complain if the results are poor.

The two advantages which a general practitioner has over the leader of a slimming club are the prestige which goes with a medical degree and the ability to prescribe slimming drugs. The former is more important, since the potency of drug treatment seems to be linked more with charisma than pharmacology (see page 136). It is significant that among the patients surveyed by Ashwell (1973) only one fifth of those who had been given slimming drugs thought they were the best way to achieve permanent weight loss, but over half said that dieting without drugs, but with the encouragement of a slimming group, was the most effective method. It is a pity, therefore, that doctors who do not want to weigh their obese patients regularly because, like Bolden (1975), they think their efforts would be better directed elsewhere, do not more readily refer their patients to slimming groups.

THE ROLE OF SLIMMING GROUPS IN THE TREATMENT OF GRADE I OBESITY

The great majority of slimming groups are sponsored by a commercial organisation, and at least one of their objectives is to make a profit from their members. It may be that the reluctance of doctors to refer patients to a slimming group comes from a desire to protect the patient from commercial exploitation. One solution is for the general practitioner to set up his own group. Craddock (1973) reports several such ventures, but does not give the results achieved. Coupar and Kennedy (1980), a clinical psychologist and general practitioner respectively, formed a non-fee-paying weight control group of 16 members with a starting weight of 81.1 ± 13.2 kg for the 9 members who subsequently attended the group, and 75.9 ± 7.7 kg for 7 who dropped out. After 10 months the attenders had an average weight loss of 6.2 kg, and by 18 months this has decreased to an average loss of 5.2 kg, while the non-attenders had on average increased weight by 2.8 kg 18 months after the start of the group.

These results are less good than those reported by Garrow (1975) and by Ashwell (1978b) for commercial slimming clubs. The average weight loss of members answering questionnaires was as follows: Weightwatchers (U.K.) 11.8 ± 7.9 kg, Slimming Magazine Club

8.6 ± 5.4 kg, Silhouette Club 7.3 ± 4.6 kg, TOPS (Take Off Pounds Sensibly) 6.6 ± 7.2 kg, and Weightwatchers (Australia) 8.2 ± 6.4 kg. However these data must be interpreted with caution: only 56.8% of members who were sent questionnaires replied, and it may be that those who did not reply were less successful than those who did. Furthermore the replies will tend to report the 'best' weight loss achieved, which is not the same as the weight loss at some arbitrary time from starting, such as 10 months, or 18 months. A truer picture would emerge if commercial slimming clubs kept a prospective record of a random sample of their membership from the time of enrollment, but, as Dwyer and Berman (1978) point out, there are several reasons why this is not likely to happen. They sent questionnaires to members of a slimming club two years after enrollment and obtained only 28% replies. These studies involve extra trouble and expense both for the organisers of the slimming club and for the members surveyed, and it is not in the commercial interests of the club that 'failures' should be documented. There is natural reluctance on the part of the members who constitute these 'failures' to fill in long questionnaires from which they can receive no benefit. If one club submitted to a thorough examination of its long-term results, and these were published, competing commercial concerns would claim better results without having to substantiate these claims.

In view of the great difficulties in getting complete unbiassed data about the performance of commercial slimming clubs the report of Seddon et al (1981) is of particular interest. In the Harrow Health District a non-profit-making slimming club was set up using local health authority premises, and with trained dietitians as group leaders. The club meets one evening per week for two hours, usually between 1930 and 2130 hrs. Members pay £6.50 (about $US 15.00 at 1980 rate of exchange) for a ten-week course, and recurrent costs are covered when there are at least 14 members in the group. The group size is limited to 30 maximum: the first 14 courses have had 249 members. The initial payment ensures the financial viability of the course, and provides an incentive for members to attend regularly. For regular attenders the total cost is less than than of commercial clubs which typically charge an enrollment fee and a weekly charge of about £1.00–1.50.

The age and obesity index of the first 249 members to enrol in the Harrow Slimming Club is shown in Figure 6.1. 43% of the membership (108/249) were grade I obese, 42% were grade II, 5% were grade III and 10% grade 0. The age distribution ranged from the teens to the seventies.

The course began and ended with a meeting run entirely by the

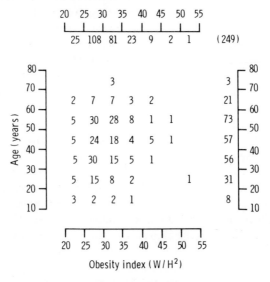

Fig. 6.1 Age (years) and obesity index (W/H^2) among 249 people who attended 10-week courses at the Harrow Slimming Club (data of Seddon et al 1981). The number of members falling in each age-W/H^2 cell is indicated, and the totals in each W/H^2 range at the upper margin, and in each age range at the right-hand margin

group leader, and the meetings 2–9 included either a film show relevant to weight loss and nutrition, or a talk by some visiting expert: physician, physiotherapist or psychologist. The attendance and weight change among members is shown in Figure 6.2. Despite the advance payment 6 of the members did not return after the first meeting, so no data about weight change are available for them. Eight members gained weight: none of these attended more than 4 sessions. The remainder showed some weight loss: the maximum loss was 25.7 kg in a man who attended every session. The average weight loss for the 243 members who attended more than one session was 4.4 kg, and it is evident from Figure 6.2 that those members who attended more sessions tended to lose more weight.

At the end of the course members who had attended at least five sessions were entitled to enrol in a follow-up course for another 10 weeks at a fee of £3.50 (about $US 8.00) at which they were weighed weekly and counselled, but no formal instruction was given. One hundred and ten took this option, and on average attended 9.2 follow-up sessions. The average weight loss during the follow-up course was 0.6 kg, ranging from a gain from the end of the main course of 6.6 kg to a further loss of 20.0 kg. There was no significant

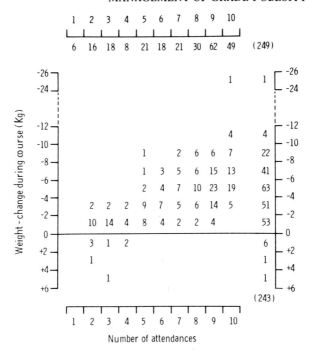

Fig. 6.2 Number of sessions attended, and weight change achieved, during a 10-week course at the Harrow Slimming Club (data of Seddon et al 1981). Layout of the figure is similar to Fig 6.1. Out of the membership of 249 there were 6 who attended only once, so no data on weight change are available. Eight attended 2–4 times, and gained weight during the course, but the remaining 235 members lost weight. Greater weight losses were observed among those who attended more regularly

relationship between the weight loss achieved on the main course and on the follow-up course. These data illustrate the great variability in response which is seen with almost any form of treatment for obesity. Some members did very well: 131 members (53%) lost more than 4 kg in 10 weeks which must be regarded as satisfactory progress. There is no reason to believe that they would have done better if they had come to a hospital clinic. At the slimming club they received 20 hours of teaching and advice in 10 weeks, and had the benefit of discussion within the group, while at hospital in 10 weeks it is unlikely that they would have spent as much as two hours in total actually talking to the doctor or dietitian. The cost to the health service of providing two hours treatment for 131 patients is very high, but at the slimming club it is virtually zero, since the subscription fee covers the hire of films and sessional payment to the dietitian. On economic grounds, therefore, the case for the slimming club system is very strong. The main argument against the slimming club is that perhaps some of the 118 members who failed to lose 4 kg in 10 weeks would have benefitted from more intensive investigation and treatment. Perhaps some of them would, particularly those who attended regularly but failed to lose much weight. In this situation the hospital can provide a back-up service to take over the management of those club members who really need to lose weight, who really try, but do not achieve weight loss.

There can be no doubt that a proper integration of non-profit-making slimming clubs with professional dietitians as group leaders, backed up by a hospital service for special cases, is a practical and economical way of providing care for the large numbers of moderately obese people in the community. The treatment of obesity inevitably involves prolonged supervision with many follow-up visits, and if these visits must be made to a hospital in normal working hours this requires a major sacrifice for people in employment or looking after small children. The locally-based slimming club is more economical for the patient, as well as for the health service. It is notable that the weight loss and attrition rate in the series reported by Seddon et al (1981) compares favourably with that reported by Stunkard and Brownell (1980) for work-site treatment of obesity. It may be that the system of a cost-covering down payment by the members, the convenient siting and timing of club meetings, and a thrifty desire to get good value for money combine to reduce the dropout rate from the slimming club.

EXERCISE IN THE PREVENTION AND TREATMENT OF OBESITY

The role of exercise in the aetiology and treatment of obesity has been greatly exaggerated by some authors. It has been suggested that obese patients should increase their daily energy expenditure by at least 1200 kcal (5 MJ) daily by taking extra exercise (Tullis 1973), that the resting metabolic rate is significantly raised for many hours after the cessation of exercise (Allen and Quigley 1977), and that moderate exercise has an anorectic effect on sedentary people (Mayer et al 1956). None of these statements is founded on good evidence. However physical activity is an important factor in maintaining fitness and energy balance, and it is right that any public health programme designed to combat obesity should lay stress on the importance of a reasonable level of physical activity.

The role of exercise in the treatment of grade I obesity will be considered under the following headings:

i. Maximal rates of energy expenditure
ii. The effect of exercise on subsequent metabolism
iii. The effect of exercise on food intake
iv. The effect of exercise on weight and body composition
v. The effect of exercise on physical fitness
vi. The role of exercise in the treatment and prevention of obesity

Maximal rates of energy expenditure

Dr Roger Bannister was particularly suited in physique, training and temperament to run the mile, and his conquest of the four-minute barrier for this event is well known. If it were possible to sustain this rate of working the marathon race (26 miles 385 yards) would be won in a time of about 1¾ hours. The original courier from the battlefield at Marathon to Athens in 490 B.C. was one Pheidippides, who fell dead on arrival. His time for the course is not known, but no modern athlete has completed the course in less than 2 hours. Champion marathon runners differ from other people in that they can sustain for 2 hours an oxygen uptake of about 4 l per minute, which is roughly equivalent to a rate of energy expenditure of 20 kcal (84 kJ) per minute. It follows that the total cost of Pheidippides fatal run was about 2500 kcal (10 MJ).

Very few people can approach the high rates of work mentioned above. Even among those people who are engaged in heavy manual labour, like workers at the coalface studied by Garry et al (1955), it is impossible to maintain an average rate of working throughout an 8 hour day above 5 kcal (20 kJ) per minute. The effect on total daily energy expenditure was that those miners who spent their working hours hacking at the rock with pickaxes used about 3660 kcal (15 MJ) per day, while men at the surface employed in clerical work used about 2800 kcal (12 MJ) per day. Thus the target of an extra 1200 kcal per day which Tullis (1973) sets his obese patients would not be met by clerical workers who did a day's work at the coalface, and it is a totally unrealistic target for obese patients.

It is a common error, when calculating the extra energy expenditure attributable to physical activity, to neglect the normal resting energy expenditure. For example a man who goes jogging for two hours at a rate of 5 kcal per minute has used 600 kcal (2.5 MJ) by the time he returns home. However if he had not gone jogging, and sat at home for the two hours, his energy expenditure would probably have been about 200 kcal (0.8 MJ) so the extra energy expenditure attributable to the jogging is only 400 kcal, not 600 kcal.

The effect of exercise on subsequent metabolism

Allen and Quigley (1977) argue that the energy cost of exercise cannot be calculated simply from the oxygen uptake during exercise, since the resting metabolic rate is significantly increased for many hours after the activity has finished. The authority for this statement is a paper by Edwards et al (1935) who were concerned to explain why the Harvard University football players needed a diet of 5,600 kcal (23 MJ) per day to maintain weight during the playing season. They made reasonable estimates of the energy cost of the actual football games and practice, and found that this figure, added to Rubner's estimate of the requirements of such men for light activity, failed to account for all the energy intake: there was about 2500 kcal (10 MJ) unaccounted for. They therefore considered the possibility that resting metabolism might be increased after exercise, and obtained some measurements consistent with, but by no means proving, this hypothesis.

In the light of newer knowledge about diet-induced thermogenesis the energy balance results of Edwards et al (1935) are less difficult to understand: certainly some of the 'missing' 2500 kcal can be ascribed to the thermogenic effect of eating 5,600 kcal per day. According to Miller and Wise (1975) there is an interaction between exercise and diet-induced thermogenesis: because these young men were both physically active and eating a large amount the thermogenic effect is enhanced. However Garby and Lammert (1977) dispute this: they found no difference in the cost of exercise with different levels of food intake on the previous day.

An important metabolic consequence of physical training is an improvement in glucose tolerance in obese patients (Sullivan 1976). Basal insulin levels are reduced, and the increase in insulin after a glucose load is also reduced, even with no alteration in the total body fat. These changes are similar to those which are observed with weight reduction in obese patients, but the mechanism by which exercise has this effect is not clear. Although a course of physical training causes a significant reduction in plasma free fatty acids and glycerol in lean subjects, this effect is not observed in obese subjects (Sullivan 1976).

The effect of exercise on food intake

Mayer et al (1954) observed that if mature adult female rats were exercised on a treadmill for progressively longer periods each day their food intake was least when they were exercising for one hour per day. Rats who exercised for longer periods ate more, as might be expected, but rats who were exercised less also showed a paradoxical increase in food intake: the difference between totally sedentary rats, and rats exercised for 1 hour was significant ($P < 0.05$). This observation gave rise to the hypothesis that regulation of food intake broke down at very low levels of physical activity, so inactivity caused obesity, not merely from a reduction in energy expenditure, but also from an increase of energy intake. This view was supported by later observations on workers in a jute mill in West Bengal (Mayer et 1956). These employees were classified into activity groups by the nature of their occupation and the distance they travelled to work. Those in very heavy jobs, like carrying bales of jute, ate most, and the lowest food intake was recorded for those classified as 'light work', namely clerks and mechanics. The critical set of observations concerned 13 stallholders, 8 supervisors and 22 clerks whose occupation was classified as 'sedentary': on average the people in these three occupations had a higher food intake, and a higher body weight, than the 'light work' group. However the stallholders and supervisors had a higher disposable income, and fewer dependents, than the clerks. It is therefore fairer to compare the food intake and body weight of 'sedentary' clerks with that of 'light work' clerks. When the analysis is done in this way the astonishing result is that sedentary clerks have a higher (reported) food intake, but a lower body weight, than 'light work' clerks.

Other studies in which the level of physical activity was altered, and the subjects were allowed to eat ad libitum, have never shown that changing from sedentary to light work was associated with a decrease in food intake (Warnold and Lenner 1977). We may conclude, therefore, that there is no acceptable evidence in man that light exercise has an anorectic effect.

The effect of exercise on weight and body composition

It may appear obvious that if obese patients are studied on a metabolic ward, on a fixed low-energy diet, they will show an accelerated rate of weight loss when an exercise programme is added to the programme of dietary restriction. In fact, this effect is very difficult to demonstrate. Figure 6.3 shows the weekly weight loss in three obese women studied by Warwick and Garrow (1981). Over a period of 14 weeks the energy expenditure of the patients was varied by exercise for 2 hours per day on a bicycle ergometer or (in one case) by raising the resting metabolic rate with a daily dose of 120 μg of triiodothyronine. There is no discernable effect of these procedures on weight loss compared with control periods without exercise or triiodothyronine. These results could be explained if the exercise was causing an increased loss of fat, with a concurrent increase in lean tissue, but the nitrogen balance data, shown in Figure 6.4, do not support this explanation. There is no difference in the trend of nitrogen balance between exercise and

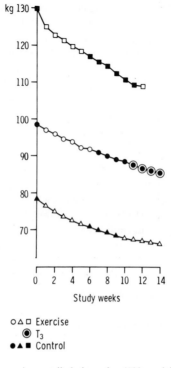

Fig. 6.3 The effect of exercise or triiodothyronine (120 μg daily) on three obese women who were given a diet supplying 3.4 MJ per day for 3 months (data of Warwick and Garrow 1981). Control, exercise and drug treatment periods are indicated by symbols. Neither the exercise not triiodothyronine affected the rate of weight loss in this study

control periods in any of the three patients, but the triiodothyronine precipitates a greatly increased nitrogen loss. Measurements of resting metabolic rate in the three patients are shown in Figure 6.5. There is no evidence that exercise affects the downward trend in metabolic rate which is to be expected on prolonged dietary restriction. The triiodothyronine causes the expected increase in resting metabolic rate.

These results are in accordance with those of Sullivan (1976) who also found that body weight and composition were not measurably affected by a programme of physical training for 35 minute sessions three days per week for 6 months. There have been reports that the effect of exercise on body weight depends on the intensity and duration of the exercise: high-intensity short-duration training tends to increase weight, while low-intensity long-duration training is associated with weight loss (Girandola 1976). It may be that the high-

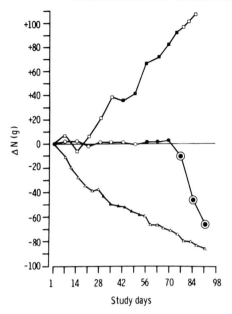

Fig. 6.4 Cumulative N balance in the three subjects shown in Fig 6.3 (data of Warwick and Garrow 1981). On a constant diet exercise did not affect N balance relative to the control period in the same subject, but triiodothyronine was associated with a greatly increased loss of lean tissue

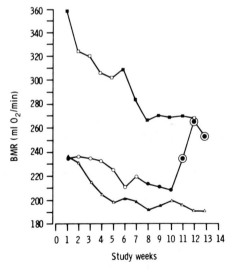

Fig. 6.5 Resting metabolic rate in the three subjects shown in Fig 6.3 (data of Warwick and Garrow 1981). Exercise had no effect on the generally decreasing metabolic rate in these subjects on a low-energy diet, but triiodothyronine caused the expected increase in resting metabolic rate

intensity training is associated with increased storage of glycogen in muscle.

The effect of exercise on physical fitness

It is beyond reasonable doubt that the performance of athletes is determined to a large degree by their level of training: this is easily documented in the laboratory by measurement of maximal oxygen uptake, and in the field by increased stamina and speed. A question of more importance to non-athletes concerns the extent to which physical training improves health in general, rather than specific athletic performance. This question is far more difficult to answer. Those who engage in regular physical activity represent a self-selected group who may be genetically different or may follow a more favourable lifestyle. It is not clear if a particular subgroup of the population would be better off in terms of life expectancy or reduced morbidity if they were to engage in running or any other specific type of physical activity (Milvy et al 1977).

Most of the information about the relationship of physical activity to health comes from epidemiological surveys. Ideally we should study large populations who are randomly allocated to high and low activity lifestyles for many years, but this is clearly impractical. A further difficulty concerns the objective measurement of the level of activity: devices are available which record physical movement (LaPorte et al 1979) but usually surveys rely on recall of daily activities (Taylor et al 1978).

A survey of 17,944 middle-aged executive grade male civil servants is reported by Chave et al (1978). They recorded leisure-time activities for two sample days in 1968–70, and their subsequent mortality was recorded over the next 10 years. Men who reported 'vigorous activity' in the survey (about 20% of the sample surveyed) suffered 1% mortality from coronary heart disease, and 4.2% from all causes during the follow-up period. The men who reported no 'vigorous activity' in the survey suffered 4.3% mortality from coronary heart disease, and 8.4% from all causes. These rates are significantly different ($P<0.01$). The definition of vigorous activity was work liable to require peaks of energy expenditure of 7.5 kcal (30 kJ) per minute or more, such as swimming, tennis, jogging or 'keep fit' exercises for at least five minutes. Men reporting activity of this sort smoked fewer cigarettes than men who did not, but the effect of activity on coronary mortality remained even when the effect of smoking was allowed for. When the general level of activity of these civil servants was related to coronary mortality there was only a weak association, which suggests that it requires fairly brisk exercise to have a protective effect. A survey of the association between activity and mortality in the Framingham population yields similar conclusions (Kannel and Sorlie 1979). More active people tend to have a lower mortality, but it is not certain if they are fit because they are active, or active because they are fit.

A mechanism by which physical activity may protect against coronary heart disease is suggested by Miller et al (1979). They note that athletes have a higher concentration of high-density lipoprotein than average, and that the greater the aerobic capacity of the athlete the higher the high-density lipoprotein concentration. The idea that exercise increases the efficiency of the heart and lungs is probably ill-founded: if only one limb or pair of limbs is trained the increased work efficiency is not seen when the untrained limbs in the same person do the work. It appears, therefore, that the effects of training occur locally in the trained muscles (Fentem 1978).

A recent study by Sedgewick et al (1980) concludes that coronary risk factors are not improved by exercise. This view is based on a series of 370 men who undertook a 12 week fitness programme, and who were examined before the training period and again 4–6 years later. There was no significant change in weight, physical working capacity, cholesterol or triglycerides. However the proponents of exercises were quick to point out that this study considered only 'risk factors' not actual coronary mortality (Moffitt 1980, Morris 1980).

The role of exercise in the prevention and treatment of moderate obesity

Before it is possible to assess the effect of exercise on obese patients it is necessary to arrange that the obese patients undertake the exercise. This is not easy. Foss et al (1976) describe a training programme for obese patients (mean $W/H^2 = 60$) based on walking measured distances on a horizontal treadmill to the point of voluntary exhaustion. At the beginning of the programme none of the 13 men and 9 women could walk two miles continuously, and only 3 (all men) could walk one mile at a speed of 1–2.5 miles per hour. Four of the patients (2 men, 2 women) never did achieve a two-mile walk, but after an average of 6 weeks training the remainder reached this goal. It is not possible from this report to judge the effect of the exercise on weight loss, because the patients were also on a strictly supervised low-energy diet.

Gwinup (1975) investigated the influence of exercise on the weight of obese subjects who were on an unrestricted diet. They were encouraged to perform regular daily exercise for an increasing period each day: most chose walking as the form of exercise. Of the 34 subjects who entered the study (29 women and 5 men) most dropped out, so data are confined to the 11 women who remained in the study. These were moderately obese (W/H² = 26.9 ± 3.7). By the end of a year of the programme 2 women were regularly walking one hour per day, 6 for two hours per day, and 3 for three hours per day. The data on weight loss are presented graphically: the average loss was 10 kg, with a range of 5–17 kg. Gwinup (1975) comments:

'Since walking produces an energy expenditure in the area of 300 kcal per hour, and since body fat contains approximately 3500 kcal per pound, it is obvious that if there had been no compensatory increase in food intake the subjects who walked for 2 hours would have been expected to lose approximately 1.25 lb/week, and those who walked for three hours, 2 lb/week. Actually, weight loss rarely exceeded 0.5 lb weekly and was usually considerably less'.

The inference that the subjects were eating more is not necessarily true, since Gwinup's calculation is based on several doubtful assumptions. The estimate of 300 kcal per hour as the energy cost of brisk walking is not unreasonable for men, but perhaps rather high for women. The assumption that those women who said they walked for two or three hours daily actually did so every day is naive, and the calculation of total energy cost falls into the trap of neglecting resting energy expenditure. Even if a subject walked for three hours at a cost of 300 kcal per hour (instead of sitting at home at a cost of 90 kcal per hour), the total energy deficit caused by the exercise is not 900 kcal, but $(3 \times 300) - (3 \times 90) = 630$ kcal. Nevertheless this study shows that highly-motivated moderately-obese people may undertake a major exercise programme and achieve a worthwhile weight loss in a year.

Lewis et al (1976) used a combination of jogging, walking, calisthenics and dietary restriction in a group of 22 moderately obese women (average W/H² = 29.4). The average weight loss was 4.2 kg in 17 weeks. They estimate that the energy cost of the entire supervised physical activity programme was about 9,100 kcal (38 MJ) which was about 19% of the total energy deficit, so the dietary restriction made a quantitatively larger contribution to the weight loss than the exercise.

Zuti and Golding (1976) compared the effect of dietary restriction, exercise, and a combination of both, on the weight and body composition of 25 moderately obese women. The study lasted 16 weeks, and each type of therapy was designed to create an energy deficit of 500 kcal (2 MJ) per day, either by reducing intake by that amount, increasing expenditure by that amount by exercise, or achieving the deficit half by energy restriction and half by extra exercise. All three treatment groups lost the same amount of weight (5 kg), but estimates of body composition, based on skinfolds and density, suggested that the exercised groups had lost more fat, and had gained lean tissue, while the dieted group had lost both fat and lean tissue. For reasons given on pages 32–34 these results must be viewed with some caution: methods for measuring changes in body composition are not accurate enough to detect the small changes reported in this paper.

Dahlkoetter et al (1979) also compared the effects of exercise, diet, and a combination of the two, on weight and physical fitness in moderately obese women. The treatment period was 8 weeks, and the weight loss achieved by the diet group was 3.2 kg, by the exercise group 2.8 kg, and by the combined group 6.1 kg. On follow-up 6 months after the end of treatment the better weight loss for the combined treatment group persisted. The exercised groups also showed considerable improvement in physical fitness, judged by the Harvard Step Test, at the end of the 8 week course. On retesting after 6 months the improvement in fitness had largely disappeared.

In summary, therefore, exercise programmes are impractical for very obese patients, but with moderately obese people they are associated with a modest weight loss, and a considerable increase in fitness. There is no convincing evidence that a programme of exercise added to dietary restriction affects the proportion of lean and fat tissue lost. Vigorous exercise in leisure time certainly is associated with lower incidence of coronary heart disease in middle-aged men: the data of Morris et al (1980) show this effect irrespective of smoking habit, stature or obesity. Even if it causes no weight loss obese patients should be encouraged to exercise.

DIET IN GRADE I OBESITY

The principles of a low-energy diet, set out on page 90, apply also to grade I obesity. However, whereas the grade III obese patient requires to lose weight urgently, the grade I obese person can afford to pursue the same objective in a more leisurely fashion. A very modest energy deficit, reflected in a very slow rate of weight loss, will do well enough. The strict application of a 'calorie counted' diet involves weighing every food item, and this is tedious. Many people prefer approximate methods which work on the principle that if certain types of food are excluded from the diet the total energy content of the diet must decrease. A survey by the Consumers' Association showed that men preferred a 'no counting' method, and women living with a family a 'low carbohydrate' method (Rudinger 1978).

The 'no counting' diet
All items of food are grouped into three categories: 'Free' foods, which can be taken in unlimited quantity; 'Restricted' foods, which can be

taken in limited quantity, and 'Forbidden' foods, which must be cut out completely.

Free foods are:

Meat, eggs, cheese, poultry (without thick sauce or stuffing)
Fish, boiled or steamed, not fried
Salads, without mayonnaise
Vegetables, cooked any way
Potatoes, not roast, fried or chip
Fresh fruit, or fruit bottled without sugar
Tea, coffee, Oxo, Bovril, Marmite, water
Condiments, Worcestershire sauce, saccharine

These foods are the important protein sources, and either have a low energy value (like fresh fruit, vegetables and salads) or else are sufficiently expensive (like meat) to prevent vast overconsumption.

The forbidden foods are:

Sugar, syrup, chocolate, sweets, cocoa, jam, honey, peanuts
Cakes, buns, biscuits, pastry, pies, tinned fruit
Spaghetti, rice, macaroni, semolina, puddings, icecream
Alcohol, sweetened fruit juice

These foods are concentrated energy sources, with relatively small contributions to essential nutrients in the diet.

The restricted foods are:

Bread, butter, margarine, breakfast cereals, milk, cream,
fats and oils.

These are staple foods which are sources of dietary fibre and of fat-soluble vitamins. Typically the allowance of bread is 3 slices (about 4 oz, or 100 g), of butter, margarine or cream 1 oz (30 g), and of milk ½ pint (300 ml) to include that taken in tea or coffee. The allowance of restricted food can be varied to achieve the desired rate of weight loss. A short alcoholic drink, or a half-pint of beer, is roughly equivalent to a slice of bread and can, if necessary, be substituted.

The advantage of this type of diet is that there are only three types of food — bread, butter and milk — which have to be taken in measured quantities: all other foods are either free or forbidden. It is therefore very easy to calculate. The disadvantage is that if the only choice of food available is 'forbidden' food the dieter must either starve or break the diet.

The 'low carbohydrate' diet

The objective of this diet is to permit the consumption of virtually any food but, by limiting carbohydrate intake, to reduce total energy intake (Yudkin 1974). To use the diet it is necessary to refer to tables published by Slimming Magazine, or in some do-it-yourself slimmers' books (Rudinger 1978, Allan 1974, Yudkin 1958). These give 'carbo-hydrate units' (CU) for items of food, each unit is equivalent to about 5 g carbohydrate. For example 1 oz (30 g) of bread is 70 kcal and 3 CU, of sugar is 110 kcal and 6 CU, of roast beef is 55 kcal and 0 CU, of butter is 225 kcal and 0 CU, and of cheddar cheese is 120 kcal and 0 CU. It is suggested that the allowance of carbohydrate should be about 50 g (10 CU) per day. For the purpose of this diet alcohol is accorded carbohydrate equivalence, so a pint (580 ml) of pale ale is 180 kcal and 9 CU, a single whisky is 50 kcal and 2½ CU, and a glass of white wine is 125 kcal and 6 CU.

The diet enables the skillful slimmer to eat a great variety of food, and whatever the fare provided by a generous host it is theoretically possible to eat something and still remain within the limits of the diet. The weakness of the diet (and to a lesser extent of the 'no counting' diet) is that the skilful slimmer can observe the restrictions but maintain a high energy intake, for example by eating large quantities of cheese, which is zero-rated for carbohydrate units. Also it promotes the idea that some foods like meat, cheese, butter and margarine are 'not fattening' despite their high energy content.

Despite these theoretical limitations these 'no counting' and 'low carbohydrate' diets are very useful for slimming groups where the advice must be easy to understand and to follow.

7

Management of grade 0 obesity

Not everyone whose weight-for-height is within the 'desirable' range is satisfied with this situation. About 10% of the members of the non-profit-making slimming club described by Seddon et al (1981) and about 13% of the membership of commerical slimming clubs (Garrow 1975) would be classified as 'grade 0' obesity, since the W/H^2 for these members falls between 20 and 25. The target weights adopted by commercial slimming clubs are around the mid-point of the desirable range: it is obviously in their economic interests to enroll members rather than reject them, and the more minimally-overweight members they have the better will be the statistics for members who achieve target weight.

There is no evidence that anyone whose W/H^2 is already below 25 will gain any benefit to health by weight loss. There may or may not be social or cosmetic benefits.

Two groups of normal-weight patients frequently seek advice about diet and weight control: those who describe themselves as 'compulsive eaters', and those who maintain normal weight by constantly eating less than what they regard as normal — these might be called 'chronic dieters'. In my experience patients in these categories are invariably female.

FEMINISM AND COMPULSIVE EATING

Orbach (1978), in a popular book entitled *Fat is a feminist issue* suggests that compulsive eating in women is a response to their social position. It is said to be the social duty of women to be attractive to men, to bear and care for children, to be the one who feeds and comforts her family and, when sacrifice is necessary, sacrifices herself. According to this ethic, fatness in a woman is evidence of greed, selfishness and a failure to fulfil her responsibilities. Brought up in this tradition, the adolescent girl may view with alarm and disgust the deposition of fat on breast, hips and thighs which is a normal part of the process of female sexual maturation. Adolescent girls who are siezed by this anxiety are candidates for anorexia nervosa: they may starve themselves in order to reverse the processes of adolescent maturation (Crisp 1973). Anorexia nervosa occurs in about 1% of all schoolgirls aged 16–18 years, but is uncommon in males (Crisp 1973).

According to Orbach (1978) the woman who survives adolescence without developing anorexia nervosa is now subjected to remorseless pressure from the advertising media that 'she must look appealing, earthy, sensual, sexual, virginal, innocent, reliable, daring, mysterious, coquettish and thin'. So unreasonable a demand naturally provokes revolt among those who do not concur with the role of women as stated above, and one way of demonstrating the rejection of these standards is to be fat.

There is undoubtedly some truth in this analysis, but its importance should not be overrated. Obesity occurs in men also, for reasons presumably unconnected with feminism, so unfeminist reasons presumably also account for some obesity in women. Although the book *Fat is a feminist issue* carries the subtitle 'How to lose weight permanently — without dieting' there is no evidence that assertion of women's right to a personality and status of their own, rather than as an adjunct to a man, has any influence on weight loss. The ethos of the feminist therapy sessions is such that the weight of members is not recorded, so there are no data on the weight loss achieved by the form of therapy which Ms Orbach offers.

Compulsive eating is not clearly defined: it is not simply eating in response to hunger, it may far exceed the amount needed to satisfy hunger, and it is always associated with feelings of protest and self-criticism. The eating binge does not bring relief from the stress which precipitated it, and the compulsive eater reports heightened anxiety during the binge, because the situation is out of control, and it is not clear what can bring it to an end. About one third of the patients coming to a hopsital obesity clinic describe episodes of compulsive eating which have terminated previous attempts to diet, especially when 'crash diets' have produced a rapid weight loss which suddenly ceased. Compulsive eating is reported in these circumstances by both men and women, but among patients at a hospital obesity clinic women outnumber men by about seven to one.

Anyone who has personal experience of a restricted diet — not necessarily a low energy diet, any diet which has an abnormally high or low content of any major nutrient — realises that prolonged dietary restriction is very annoying, and whatever type of food is forbidden on the diet becomes unreasonably attractive. One does not have to invoke feminist concepts to explain the tensions which arise when a young woman of normal weight struggles unsuccessfully to force her weight to a still lower level in order to achieve a more acceptable figure. Non-existant obesity (or even genuine obesity) is often used as a whipping-boy for all sorts of dissatisfaction with social success: if only he or she were thin, then .... The supposed consequences of thinness are often highly improbable, especially in a grade 0 obese person who is only trying to lose a few pounds.

It is clearly inappropriate to give the normal-weight compulsive eater advice on a reducing diet, and still worse to prescribe anorectic drugs. It is important to try to find out why this person is trying to lose weight, what they would regard as an ideal weight, and what they expect to be able to do at this ideal weight which they cannot do now. Often patients have never formulated answers to these questions, and when they do so it provides some insight into their problem. When these questions are posed patients often keep returning to some alarming experience of weight gain which they fear will recur unless they are vigilant: having dieted for two weeks they put back all the weight they had lost in a single weekend. This experience is generalised to the conclusion that to maintain weight they can only eat 'normally' for two days in fourteen.

In this situation reassurance may help, backed by some scientific evidence. Yes, it is possible to gain one or two kilogrammes in one or two days by suddenly repleting glycogen stores (see page 20) but it is quite impossible to gain fat at the rate of a kilogramme per day, since this would require an excess of intake over expenditure of more than 9000 kcal (38 MJ). In the long run weight can be maintained if, and only if, energy input matches energy output. The truth of these statements can, if necessary, be demonstrated in a metabolic ward, but it is impractical to use such expensive facilities simply to allay the anxiety of normal-weight people about their metabolism. Indeed, it is difficult to judge how much time and effort it is reasonable to invest in treating normal-weight people who express anxiety about obesity. At least they are entitled to a reasonable explanation of the phenomena which worry them, but if they do not find the explanation satisfying a commitment to a deeper analysis of the problem is very time-consuming. Perhaps group therapy sessions of the type described by Orbach (1978) is the best solution.

THE NORMAL-WEIGHT 'CHRONIC DIETER'

The person who, in order to maintain normal weight, must constantly restrict food intake deserves sympathy and encouragement. Often, they do not get it. In the survey of Ashwell (1973) of patients who had consulted their general practitioners about obesity 9% say that they were told not to worry about their weight. Whether these people were, or were not, overweight it should have been possible to give more helpful advice than this.

Consider the situation of a person who weighed 80 kg, ate 2800 kcal (12 MJ) per day, and was gaining weight. So far as that person is concerned 2800 kcal is a normal intake. Suppose this person loses 15 kg over a period of a year by conscientious dieting, and having reached 65 kg considers it is reasonable now to eat 'normally'. Obviously since 'normal' eating caused weight gain at 80 kg it will cause even more rapid weight gain at 65 kg, when the resting oxygen uptake will be about 20 ml/minute less than it was before weight loss (Doré et al 1981). Inevitably, therefore, formerly obese people regard the diet on which they can maintain weight after substantial weight loss as restrictive.

Often the situation is further complicated by the incomplete fulfilment of the expected benefits of weight loss. Bruch (1974) has an excellent chapter on what she calls 'thin fat people' — formerly obese people who need the help of a psychiatrist because they find that the Promised Land of slimness does not come up to expectations. She cites the example of Beryl, a young woman who had reduced her weight from 114 kg to 61 kg and thereby gained the approval of her father. Although she now looked beautiful she was not satisfied:

'I want to be underweight so I can stop worrying about what I eat. I still cannot eat sweets like ordinary people. The minute I eat sweets my system craves a lot. I have to do one or the other, either diet — or go hog wild on sweets and all that stuff'.

Her ambition to be so slim that she can eat sweets in unlimited quantity can never be fulfilled. She is already as slim as she can reasonably be, and however much she starved it would merely serve to reduce her metabolic requirements still further. Whatever benefits weight loss may bring, the ability to eat ad libitum without weight gain cannot be one of them.

This being so, was the effort to lose weight worthwhile? Usually the answer is Yes. People forget the disadvantages of obesity when they become thin. It is not as if the person who has reduced in weight has exchanged a carefree existence as a fat person for the tyranny of perpetual dieting. Even as a fat person it was not possible to eat unlimited sweets with impunity, and there were other disadvantages as well. Probably a psychiatrist such as Bruch sees a higher proportion of formerly obese patients who had totally unrealistic ideas about the benefits of weight loss, and who consequently suffered greater-than-average psychological trauma when these expectations were not fulfilled.

'Fat people are apt to blame all their difficulties on being fat and they hope for a new lease on life after they get thin' (Bruch 1974). It is the responsibility of the therapist not only to guide the patient honestly about the means to achieve weight loss, but also about the realistic consequences of weight loss for that particular patient. The items which can reasonably be included in the prospectus are discussed in Chapter 2: weight loss is usually a good bargain, but it should not be over-sold, or the therapist will lay up trouble for both himself and the patient in the future.

8

The management of obesity in pregnant women

The dietary management of pregnant women is a subject on which many obstetricians have strong views. There is good epidemiological evidence that fetal growth is impaired in women of lower socio-economic groups. One of the respects in which these women differ from more affluent women is a lower plane of nutrition. There is ample evidence from, for example, pig farmers that very well-fed sows produce heavier and healthier piglets. On this basis Brewer (1967) says that it is mandatory that pregnant women should be given truly heroic quantities of food, especially protein. He ascribes growth failure in the fetus largely to maternal malnutrition. If we adopt this view there can be no question of attempting to treat obesity during pregnancy.

Craddock (1973) adopts a different attitude:

'The six month period during which a pregnant woman attends for antenatal supervision affords the physician the chance of practising true preventive medicine, the like of which is hard to equal in the whole field of patient/doctor contact in the western world.'

He feels that if the pregnant woman is obese this is an opportunity to control the situation, at least by limiting weight gain during pregnancy. Hytten (1979) takes a characteristically cool view. He notes that attempts to control pre-eclamptic toxaemia by dietary restriction have failed, and does not expect attempts to control obesity to do much better. He concedes that there may be a case for intervention in grossly obese women, but 'to attempt reduction of food intake when the woman is having a surge of appetite is swimming against the tide ...'. It may be quite sensible to try to swim against the tide if the alternative — drifting with the tide — is very likely to land you in trouble.

NUTRIENT REQUIREMENTS IN PREGNANCY

The recommended daily energy intake for groups of pregnant women in the U.K. (Department of Health and Social Security 1979) and in the United States (National Academy of Sciences and National Research Council 1964) agree in suggesting an extra 200 kcal (0.8 MJ) daily above non-pregnant requirements. The recommended intake of protein is increased from 54 g to 60 g per day, of calcium from 500 mg to 1200 mg per day, and the pregnant woman is recommended to take 10 μg cholecalciferol per day. There are small upward adjustments in the recommended intake of other vitamins and iron.

The energy requirements of mature pregnant and lactating women have been measured by Blackburn and Calloway (1976) who obtained estimates of 2260 kcal (9.5 MJ), 2520 kcal (10.5 MJ), and 2600 kcal (10.9 MJ) for the periods of gestation 20–28 weeks, 29–36 weeks, and 37–40 weeks respectively. These values were calculated on the assumption that the energy cost of weight gain was 146 kcal (0.61 MJ) per day between 20–28 weeks, and 243 kcal (1.02 MJ) thereafter. Energy requirements for lactating women were calculated at 2530 kcal (10.6 MJ) per day, assuming the energy cost of milk secretion was 675 kcal (2.8 MJ) per day.

THE EFFECT OF PREGNANCY ON BODY WEIGHT AND COMPOSITION

The weight gain during a normal pregnancy averages about 12.5 kg. In their classic review Hytten and Leitch (1964) calculate that 7 kg of this is water, about 0.9 kg is protein of which half is in the fetus, and about 4 kg of fat are added to the mother's energy stores, as a reserve to support lactation.

The measurements of Pipe et al (1979) agree with these estimates: they found that of a weight gain of 10.4 kg between 12 and 37 weeks of pregnancy 7.2 kg could be accounted for as water. The increase in fat stores occurs mainly during the first trimester of pregnancy, and a modest increase in the lean tissues of the mother — about 0.9 kg —occurs in the last two trimesters. In the patients studied by Pipe et al (1979) body weight and composition returned almost exactly to the values at 10–14 weeks gestation within 6–15 weeks of delivery of the baby.

This return to pre-pregnancy weight is the crucial point concerning the importance of pregnancy to subsequent obesity. Hytten (1979) says that there is a trend for women to become heavier with increasing age, but that parity makes a negligible contribution to this weight increase. The best data on this point are those of Billewicz and Thomson (1970). They compared the weight at 20 weeks gestation in a first pregnancy with the weight at 20 weeks gestation in subsequent pregnancies in a large series of women in Aberdeen. On average, having allowed for the expected increase in weight with time, the weight increase from first to second pregnancies was 1 kg, from first to third was 1.5 kg, and from first to fourth 1.9 kg. These weight increases are indeed small on average, but a minority of women gained an unusually large amount of weight with parity. The mean weight gain among women who were initially underweight was only 0.8 kg, but those who were initially overweight gained an average of 2.4 kg. Furthermore, those women who gained most weight between pregnancies tended to gain most during pregnancies.

Similar conclusions can be derived from the data of Beazley and Swinhoe (1979), which are illustrated in Fig 8.1. They followed the weight change of 50 women in Liverpool through five successive pregnancies. For the first 3 pregnancies, weight 6 weeks post-partum had fallen below weight at the 20th of pregnancy, but for the fourth and fifth pregnancies this was no longer so. Weight gain tended to be greatest among those who were heaviest: the average weight of the whole series increased by 5.1 kg between the 20th week of the first and fifth pregnancy (from 59.1 kg to 64.2 kg), but the heaviest quartile of mothers increased 7.83 kg (from 73.02 kg to 80.85 kg). Thus, while it may be fair to say that, for the population as a whole, pregnancy has only a small effect on weight gain, there is a section of the population, who are already the most overweight, in whom pregnancy is associated with a much greater weight gain.

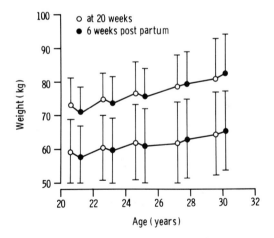

Fig. 8.1 Weight change between 20 weeks gestation and 6 weeks post partum in 50 women followed through five successive pregnancies (data of Beazley and Swinhoe 1979). The lower line shows the Mean ± S.E.M. weight for the whole series, and the upper line for the heaviest quartile of mothers. The tendency for post-partum weight to be less than weight at 20 weeks gestation disappears after the third pregnancy

THE EFFECT OF OBESITY ON REPRODUCTIVE PERFORMANCE

Menstrual irregularity is a common complaint among obese women. Combes et al (1979) observed irregular cycles in 47% of a series of 231 obese women, but in only 25% of a control series of normal-weight women of the same age. Hartz et al (1979) analysed questionnaires from 73,532 members of the TOPS organization and concluded that the more obese women were more likely to have irregular or anovulatory cycles, and were more likely to be infertile.

When pregnant, obese women are more likely to suffer complications of pregnancy. Peckham and Christianson (1971) selected a series of light, medium and heavy women, matched for height, with 394 women in each weight group. The incidence of toxaemia and of hypertension was 7.9% and 6.4% in the heavy group, compared with 0.3% and 2.0% in the light group. Among primiparae the mean duration of labour was 13.26 hours in the heavy group, and 11.24 hours in the light group. Edwards et al (1978) compared the outcome of pregnancy among 208 obese women with that of lean controls matched for age, parity and race. They found the obese mothers had a higher incidence of hypertension and gestational diabetes (P<0.05). Efiong (1975) compared 100 pregnant women who weighed over 80 kg at the 14th week of pregnancy with a control series, matched for height, age, parity and social class, who weighed less than 65 kg. The heavier group of women had more complications in pregnancy, notably hypertension, pre-eclampsia, glycosuria and pyelitis of pregnancy. There were two maternal deaths, both in the heavy group. Maeder et al (1975) also note the danger to the mother of obesity. They analysed a series of 250 maternal deaths and showed that 41% of the mothers who died weighed more than 150 lb (68 kg) and 12% more than 200 lb (91 kg). In a control series only 15% exceeded 150 lb and 2% exceeded 200 lb.

Thus there is ample evidence that obesity is a disadvantage to the pregnant woman.

MATERNAL WEIGHT GAIN AND THE OUTCOME OF PREGNANCY

It is well established that, in general, a weight gain of about 12.5 kg during pregnancy is associated with the minimum perinatal mortality (Hytten 1980). Obstetricians regard steady weight gain as a sign that the pregnancy is going normally. The question which concerns us is if this general rule applies also to women who are already overweight when they begin their pregnancy — should they ideally gain another 12.5 kg, or should they finance some of the energy cost of pregnancy from their excess stores of body fat?

In the United States, between 1959 and 1966, a massive prospective study was set up to follow the outcome of 53,518 pregnancies. With so large a data base it is possible to divide the whole series into many subgroups, and thus to compare the outcome of pregnancy in overweight and underweight mothers, and in each weight group those who gained a large or small amount of weight during pregnancy. This valuable analysis has been published by Naeye (1979). Having excluded all twins, pregnancies which lasted less than 20 weeks, cases in which the mother's pre-pregnancy weight or height were not known, mothers with active tuberculosis, organic heart disease, severe anaemia, diabetes mellitus, alcoholism or drug addiction, there remained 44,565 pregnancies suitable for analysis. The pre-pregnancy weight of the mothers was divided into four categories according to their weight as a percentage of the Metropolitan Life Insurance Company Ideal weight for 'medium frame' women of the same height. It is more convenient to convert these into W/H^2 notation: 11% of the mothers were underweight (W/H^2 less than 19), 51% were desirable weight (W/H^2) 19–22.9), 28% were mildly overweight (W/H^2 23–28), and 10% were definitely overweight (W/H^2 greater than 28). The weight gain during pregnancy was divided into five categories by expressing the mother's weight gain as a percentage of the 'optimal' rate of weight gain. For purposes of this analysis the optimal gain was assumed to be 8.5 lb (3.9 kg) at 20 weeks, 19 lb (8.6 kg) at 30 weeks, and 27 lb (12.3 kg) at 40 weeks.

Figure 8.2 shows that among mothers of 'desirable' weight 41% gained weight at a rate between 80% and 120% of the 'optimal' rate. Very few (3%) gained at less than 25% of the optimal rate, and 14% gained at more than 120% of the optimal rate. Similar rates of weight gain were seen in the underweight mothers. However, with the mildly overweight and definitely overweight mothers less-than-optimal weight gains were commoner. All four maternal weight groups showed similar proportions of mothers with more-than-optimal rates of weight gain during pregnancy.

It is implicit in the idea of 'optimal' weight gain that mothers who depart from this rate of weight gain should fare worse than those who conform to it. So far as desirable-weight and under-weight mothers this expectation is fulfilled: perinatal mortality rates were lowest among those mothers whose weight gain was within 20% of 'optimal'. However, the more overweight the mother the lower the perinatal mortality at lower rates of weight gain: these results are ilustrated in

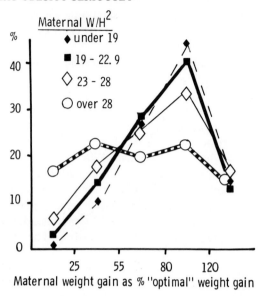

Fig. 8.2 Weight gain during pregnancy related to the pre-pregnancy weight status of the mother (recalculated from the data of Naeye 1979, based on 44,565 pregnancies). The weight gain during pregnancy is expressed as % of 'optimal' weight gain, assumed to be 27 lb (12.3 kg) at 40 weeks gestation. The pre-pregnancy weight of the mother has been recalculated as W/H^2. About 15% of mothers gain more than 120% of 'optimal' weight, whatever their previous weight status, but very small weight gains are more commonly observed among the more overweight mothers.

Figure 8.3. With definitely overweight mothers the 'optimal' rate of weight gain was no longer associated with minimum mortality: those who gained only about 7 kg (16 lb) had a lower perinatal mortality rate (30.8 deaths per 1000 births) than those who gained the 'optimal' amount (35.0 deaths per 1000 births).

This study provides a definitive answer to the question posed at the beginning of this section: in terms of perinatal mortality there seems to be no advantage — indeed a slight disadvantage — in encouraging the overweight mother to gain the normal 12.5 kg during pregnancy. From the viewpoint of the subsequent health of the mother there is every advantage in trying to restrict the weight gain of the overweight pregnant woman to about half the normal amount. The evidence therefore supports the view of Craddock (1973) that pregnancy presents a golden opportunity for nutritional counselling, not only with respect to the control of obesity in pregnancy, but also to show the mother how she can influence the health of herself and her family by

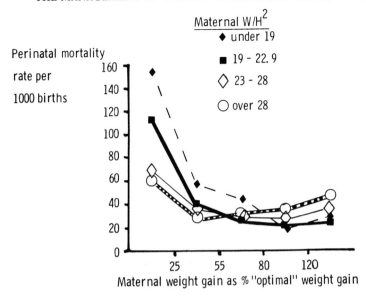

Fig. 8.3 Perinatal mortality related to maternal weight gain (data of Naeue 1979). Among normal-weight or underweight mothers perinatal mortality is least with 'optimal' weight gain, but overweight mothers show a lower perinatal mortality with about half the 'optimal' weight gain in pregnancy

the appropriate choice of diet. If the obstetrician neglects to take this opportunity he really cannot expect that the patient's obesity will have been magically cured by someone else before the next pregnancy begins.

THE EFFECT OF DIETARY RESTRICTION IN HUMAN PREGNANCY

Even if it is accepted, on the basis of the evidence on pp. 175–177, that the perinatal mortality in overweight mothers is better at about half the normal rate of weight gain, two practical problems remain. First, as mentioned by Hytten (1979), there is the problem of getting the mother to eat less at a time when her appetite is increasing, and second, there is the question of effects on subsequent development of the child. Perinatal mortality is rather a crude index of the success of pregnancy if the children survive, but do not develop normally.

It is certainly possible, by dietary advice, to restrict the weight gain of pregnant women to about half of that shown by similar women eating to appetite. A series published by Borberg et al (1980) demonstrates this point: thin, normal-weight and obese women eating to appetite gained 12.9 kg, 11.9 kg and 13.6 kg respectively between 16 weeks gestation and delivery, and after delivery they weighed 6.3 kg, 2.8 kg and 4.9 kg more than their weight at 16 weeks gestation. However a group of obese women who were advised to take a diet which provided 150–180 g carbohydrate, and about 1800–2000 kcal, gained only 6.2 kg between 16 weeks gestation and delivery, and after delivery they weighed on average 2.3 kg less than their weight at 16 weeks. Thus quite a modest degree of dietary restriction can achieve the restriction in weight gain which the data of Naeye (1979) suggest is best for the overweight mother. Borberg et al (1980) observe that the impairment of glucose tolerance, which is a feature both of pregnancy and of obesity, can be ameliorated by this type of dietary restriction, and that there was no adverse effect on neonatal outcome.

Concerning the possible effects of dietary restriction during pregnancy on the subsequent development of the child it is less easy to obtain hard evidence. Obviously development is influenced by many factors other than intra-uterine nutrition, so it is difficult to attribute developmental handicap in later life to any particular perinatal factor. One piece of evidence which was thought to indicate that intra-uterine nutrition affected mental development was derived by intelligence testing of twins. Twins have a lower birthweight than singleton babies, and they tend to score lower in intelligence tests than singleton babies matched for social class. This might indicate that the twin, who had to share the available intra-uterine nutrition, suffered a permanent setback to mental development.

The fallacy of this conclusion was shown by McKeown (1970). He compared the score of twins with singleton children in the '11-plus' examination, designed to select children for academic secondary schooling, and found that they scored lower, as expected. However when children were chosen who were single survivors of twin pregnancies the difference from singleton pregnancies vanished. This strongly suggests that the poorer score of twins was largely due to post-natal factors, and not to the level of intrauterine nutrition.

There is much epidemiological evidence of mental impairment in children living in poor social circumstances, but it is impossible to dissect away nutritional factors from those connected with genetic endowment and environmental factors such as the level of intellectual stimulation of the child. From the scientific viewpoint we need a randomly selected sample of population who are subjected to severe dietary restriction in an otherwise affluent community. This is obviously ethically impossible as a scientific experiment, but something very near to this experiment happened inadvertently in Holland during the winter of 1944–1945. The Allied forces entered the

Netherlands on September 14th 1944, and planned to sieze the bridges at Arnhem and Nijmegen, which were the key to the cities of the north-west — The Hague, Amsterdam and Rotterdam. To hamper the German defence of this territory the Dutch government-in-exile in London broadcast an appeal to resistance workers to sabotage the transport system, while an airborne unit tried to take the bridges. The transport strike was successful, but the paratroop raid was not, so by mid-November 1944 the Allied forces had liberated the Netherlands south of the Rhine, but the north-west coastal cities were completely cut off from their sources of food supply. That winter was exceptionally severe, and there were no stocks of food, so until May 7th, 1945 there was famine in north-west Holland, but relatively normal food supply in the south of the country.

The effect of this famine on the development of children born before, during and after the hungry winter has been carefully documented by Stein et al (1975) in one of the classic studies of human undernutrition. It was possible to compare children born in the blockaded zone with those born at the same time in parts of the country where there was adequate food. If, as Brewer (1967) suggests, maternal malnutrition leads to fetal malnutrition, there should have been no difficulty in demonstrating the fact in the children born in the famine area, but the only striking finding was that the starved women ceased to menstruate. This seems to be the defence of the human species against famine: women become infertile — but once a pregnancy is established in a reasonably well-nourished mother the fetus does not go short. Compared with the young of other species the human baby is unusually small and slow-growing, so it presents a far smaller nutritional burden on the mother. As Hytten (1980) puts it:

'The point to be made here is that, within wide limits, the fetus of a reasonably healthy, pregnant woman is remarkably unaffected by dietary inadequacy during pregnancy and is difficult to damage by overall restriction of food'.

This is not a licence to ignore the nutritional requirements of pregnancy (see pp. 171–172) but it does give the obstetrician an opportunity to control obesity in pregnancy to the advantage of both the mother and her child.

The effect of maternal diet on lactational performance is not clear. Blackburn and Calloway (1976) calculate that the energy cost of lactation is 675 kcal (2.8 MJ) per day, and maternal fat stores, laid down during pregnancy, will normally supply this energy (Hytten and Leitch 1964). If the diet has been restricted during pregnancy this probably does not affect lactation. In Gambian mothers an energy supplement increased the weight of the mothers, but did not affect the volume or fat content of their milk (Prentice et al 1980).

9

The management of obesity in childhood

The management of an obese child is an important but difficult task. It is just as important, and not quite so difficult, to use the child health monitoring organisations to steer potentially obese children away from the path which leads to obesity in adult life. The aim is to regulate the energy intake of the child to a level which supports normal growth and development, as indicated by centile lines on the paediatric growth charts. This objective is made more difficult to attain because the diet of a child is regulated by the mother and often many other people —father, grandparents, child-minder, school meals organiser — who may have all sorts of selfish or altruistic motives for overfeeding the child, or who may merely be unaware that there is a problem with the child's weight.

ASSESSMENT AND INVESTIGATION OF OBESITY IN CHILDHOOD

In adults it is possible, without significant error, to define obesity in terms of the index W/H^2 (see pages 3 and 27). With children there is no numerical index which is satisfactory (Newens and Goldstein 1972), since during development weight and height accelerate at different rates. Around puberty the situation is very complex, and purist anthropometrists cannot define the limits of normal weight in pre-pubertal children except retrospectively, in the light of knowledge of the age at puberty.

The measures of obesity in children which are practically useful are charts which indicate centile range for height and weight against age, and skinfold measurements. Hormonal or genetic causes of obesity are almost invariably associated with short stature. It is important to make the diagnosis if a child is hypothyroid or has an inborn error of metabolism, but it is also important not to subject the child to a series of uninformative investigations for which there is no clinical indication. Parents are often convinced that their offspring 'must have some glandular problem', and an elaborate series of investigations (even if the results are negative) tends to support the view that this is a theory worth testing. If the child is above-average height for age (as obese children often are) it is very unlikely that there is a metabolic disease underlying the obesity, and requests for investigations should be resisted as far as possible. If the parents insist, and are obviously unwilling to listen to any dietary advice until the tests have been done, then X-rays for pituitary fossa and for bone age, a blood count and measurement of plasma urea, electrolytes and thyroid hormones is a reasonably thorough and non-traumatic set of investigations.

If a child is of short stature and obese these tests should be done with as little fuss as possible: it is important that the parents should not have the idea implanted that their child is metabolically abnormal, or their attentions will be deflected from the task of dietary management.

Measurements of skinfold thickness at eight sites (Udal et al 1976) are particularly useful in assessing obesity in new-born infants. However measurement technique affects the answers which are obtained so each investigator needs to set up his own standards within his series. Centile values for triceps skinfolds in American whites are shown in Figures 9.1 and 9.2 (data of Garn and Clark, 1976). The values for boys and girls are similar for the first six years of life, but the increase in fat before puberty is greater, and starts earlier, in girls than in boys.

To measure the triceps skinfold the subject should be seated with the arm flexed at the elbow and the forearm supported, so the muscles of the upper arm are relaxed. A point is marked midway between the acromion and olecranon processes in the mid-posterior line of the arm. With the forefinger and thumb of the left hand applied about 5 cm

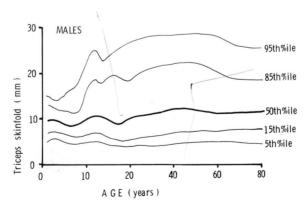

Fig. 9.1 Centile values for triceps skinfold thickness in white American males (data of Garn and Clark 1976)

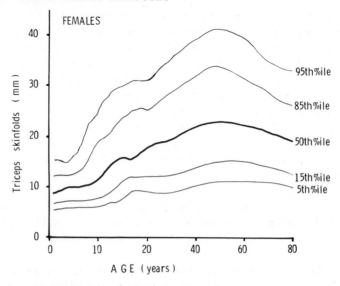

Fig. 9.2 Centile values for triceps skinfold thickness in white American females (data of Garn and Clark 1976)

above this mark a fold of skin and underlying fat is picked up, so the long axis of the fold is in line with the humerus, and skinfold calipers are applied at the marked point. The calipers (Harpenden) are spring-loaded so the measuring faces apply a constant pressure: the handle of the caliper must be released so this pressure is applied to the skin. In new-born babies it is particularly important to leave the calipers in place for 60 seconds before taking the reading, because the skin of young babies is often oedematous, and tends to give too high a reading at first (Whitelaw 1976). The procedure should be repeated on the other arm to ensure that it is reproducible.

CRITICAL PERIODS AND FAT CELL NUMBER

The fat cell hypothesis of Hirsch (1975) was that

'obesity may be accompanied by an excessive number of adipocytes, possibly brought about by excessive feeding in infancy and childhood, and that this excessive number of adipocytes remains constant and in some way causes a drive for maintaining the obese state'.

This hypothesis has given rise to much controversy and research, since, if it is true, it is particularly important that infants should not be overfed. To understand the current research in this field it is necessary to appreciate the difficulties in measuring fat cell number.

Techniques for measuring total fat cell number

Hirsch and Gallian (1968) developed a technique for taking needle biopsy samples of subcutaneous adipose tissue and fixing the fat cells in osmium tetroxide. The sample was then crumbled, sieved, and the number of particles was electronically counted. If these particles are assumed to represent the number of fat cells in the original sample, and if the total amount of fat in an aliquot of the sample has been determined, it is possible to estimate the average amount of fat per fat cell. Suppose this is 0.4 μg of fat per cell, and the subject from whom the sample came had 12 kg of fat, then the number of fat cells can be calculated:

$$\text{Fat cell number} = \frac{\text{total body fat (g)}}{\text{average fat per cell (g)}} = \frac{12 \times 10^3}{4 + 10^{-7}} = 3 \times 10^{10}$$

The problems in measuring total body fat have been discussed (see pp. 29–34). Even greater problems arise from the assumption that the particles reflect the number of fat cells in the sample, and that the fat cell size in the sample is representative of the fat cell size throughout the body.

The original osmium tetroxide method is not generally used today, because it fails to detect very small fat cells, and hence underestimates fat call number in the sample, hence overestimates fat cell size and underestimates fat cell number in the whole body. Histological techniques are quicker, more sensitive, and do not involve such toxic reagents. However it is likely that there are connective tissue cells in the body which are capable of storing fat if necessary, but which may contain no fat at the time when the fat biopsy is taken (Ashwell 1978a). If there are 'preadipocytes' they will not be detected by any available method for counting fat cells, since these depend on the fat content of the cell to recognise an adipocyte (Gurr and Kirtland 1978a, b).

The idea that samples of subcutaneous adipose tissue yield a true estimate of fat cell size is disputed by Jung et al (1978) who point out that intra-abdominal fat cells are usually smaller than subcutaneous fat cells, and that with fat gain and loss the ratio of subcutaneous to intra-abdominal fat may change.

Age of onset of obesity and fat cell number

The hypothesis put forward by Hirsch (1975) was based on the observation that the most obese patients tended to have become obese during childhood, and they also had the largest apparent fat cell number. However it is now agreed that if people with similar amounts of fat are compared, there is no significant relationship between the fat cell number and the age of onset (Hirsch and Batchelor 1976, Ashwell 1979). It is tempting to postulate that during early life fat cells multiply in number, and later increase in size, but this does not seem to be the normal course of development in most tissues (Sands et al 1979). Knittle et al (1977) have made serial measurements of fat cell size in obese and non-obese children. They report a steep increase in apparent fat cell number at about age 10 in obese children, but since these measurements were made with the osmium tetroxide method this may simply mean that in these children more cells had accumulated enough fat to be detected.

Krotkiewski et al (1977) classified a group of 90 obese women into four groups on the basis of their adipose tissue cellularity: borderline, hypertrophic, hyperplastic and combined. The hypertrophic group had a normal number of large fat cells, the hyperplastic had a large number of normal-sized cells, and the combined group a large number of large fat cells. This combined group were the most obese, had the earliest onset of obesity, lost most weight on treatment and regained it most rapidly. The authors ascribe the relapse rate to the high fat cell number, but it is not clear how a high fat cell number causes obesity to persist. It might be that people with many fat cells experienced greater hunger on a reducing diet, but this does not seem to be so (Durrant and Ashwell 1979). Alternatively people with obesity of early onset might have particularly low metabolic rates, but again the evidence does not support this view (Garrow et al 1980).

AETIOLOGY OF CHILDHOOD OBESITY

Genetic factors in childhood obesity

In some strains of rodent, such as the Zucker rat, obesity is genetically determined. Although it can be modified by feeding the tendency to obesity still emerges (Johnson et al 1973). Genetic factors certainly influence the pattern of deposition of fat in children: monozygotic twins have more similar skinfold measurements than dizygotic twins (Brook et al 1975, Borjeson 1976) and the skinfolds of newborn babies of obese mothers are thicker than babies of thin mothers (Whitelaw 1976, Udall et al 1978). It may be that some families have a 'thrifty gene' (Neel 1962) but it is a mistake to assume that characteristics shared by families are necessarily genetically determined (Garn and Clark 1976): fat dog-owners tend to have fat dogs (Mason 1970) but in this case the explanation is obviously not genetic.

The findings from the Ten-State Nutrition Survey may be interpreted to support or refute the idea that genetic factors are important in determining obesity in children. Since more than 40,000 people were examined it is possible to trace obesity through family lines, with many parental and sibling fatness combinations (Garn and Clark 1976). If parents and children are classified as lean if they are below the 15th centile in skinfold thickness, obese if they are above the 85th centile, and medium if they are between these limits, it is possible to calculate the correlation between fatness in parents and fatness in their children. On average the children of two lean parents were leanest, and those of two obese parents were fattest, with intermediate parental combinations producing children of intermediate fatness. Children with one lean and one obese parent were of similar fatness to those of parents who were both of medium fatness. It made little difference if it was the father or mother who was obese, nor were correlations of fatness significantly stronger for parents and children of the same sex than of the opposite sex.

This result is certainly compatible with the view that genetic influences are important, although it does not indicate any particular pattern of inheritance. However there are two findings from this large study which cast serious doubt on the importance of genetic influences. Analysis of similarities in fatness between spouses shows correlation as strong as that found between parents and children, which increased with time. This cannot be due to genetic influences, since spouses are not genetically similar, but presumably reflects the effect of family attitudes to food and weight. These attitudes would apply also to the children of the marriage, so it suggests that some, and perhaps most, of the parent-child similarity in fatness is due to environmental rather than genetic influences.

Another observation from the Ten-State Nutrition Survey which weakens the case for genetic determination of obesity concerns the relationship of social class to obesity. It has been well established that obesity is commoner among the lower socioeconomic groups (see page 186) which is not in itself an argument against genetic influences. It might be that genes associated with obesity occur unevenly across the social spectrum. However, in prepubertal girls, those of the lower socioeconomic classes are leaner than those of more affluent parents, but at puberty the situation is reversed. Furthermore the influence of social class on obesity is stronger with women than with men. These findings are easier to explain on the basis of environmental influences than on the basis of heredity.

The argument about the contribution of genetic factors to predisposition to obesity will never be finally settled until we have some unequivocal genetic marker, like a blood group or cell type, which can be shown to be linked to the obese tendency. We have no such marker in man, and probably never will have. In the light of the available evidence it is not possible to take the view that genetic influences are very important in determining human obesity, since it is so easy to find examples which do not fit the hypothesis, and to find alternative explanations in those cases which seem to support the hypothesis.

Social factors in childhood obesity

Bruch (1940) pioneered the idea that obesity in children was a manifestation of social problems in the family. In the 1930s the idea of endocrine causes of obesity was dominant, and the diagnosis of Frölich's syndrome was made in fat children with delayed sexual development. Bruch pointed out that they were overfed and overprotected; in a series of 142 obese children 35% were only children and a further 35% were youngest in the family.

It may be that in the children referred to Bruch, as a child psychiatrist, psychological problems were over-represented, but no experienced clinician would deny that the problems of an obese child are much more likely to arise from relationships within the family than from a lesion in the pituitary gland. Hammar et al (1972) studied 10 obese and 10 non-obese adolescents and found that the obese girls had an earlier menarche, but a normal growth hormone response to insulin and normal thyroid function. The obese differed from the non-obese in having more parental conflicts, more feeding problems, were more often given sweets as bribes, and had lower self-esteem. Bruch (1961) suggests that normal mechanisms of hunger and satiety will never develop in a child who is fed for all sorts of reasons other than the need for food: if, whenever the child is in an emotional crisis, sweets are offered as a comfort, it is not surprising if the child comes to regard food as an appropriate solution to emotional crises, rather than something you take when hungry.

It is not only the child who has an emotional need for food. It is the role of the mother to feed her family, and it causes greater distress to many women to restrict the food of a child than to restrict their own food intake, even though they accept that it is in the interests of the child to eat less. Obese adults coming as patients to a hospital obesity clinic may give as a reason for being unable to diet themselves the excuse that they have to provide food for their family, even though they may agree that all the family could benefit from weight loss.

The strong negative association between obesity and social class (Stunkard 1975) which is reversed in prepubescent girls (Garn and Clark 1976) is also evidence of the relevance of the social environment to obesity, but the reason for this association is not clear. A survey by

Ashwell and Etchell (1974) found that the higher prevalence of obesity among people in the lower socioeconomic strata could not be explained on the hypothesis that such people did not know, or did not care, that they were overweight.

As with so many theories about the aetiology of childhood obesity, it is easy to overstate the importance of environmental factors. A study by Dubois et al (1979) found rather modest differences between the feeding practices of the mothers of 47 obese infants and 42 normal infants. It is not true that obese infants are never breast fed or differ markedly in the time at which solid food is introduced. It would be astonishing if there were clear-cut differences between obese and normal weight children in these respects, since obese infants do not always remain obese, nor do thin always remain thin.

DO FAT BABIES STAY FAT?

The main importance of obesity in childhood lies in its long-term effects. If it is true that fat children become fat adults then childhood is the obvious time at which to try to prevent adult obesity. But what are the chances that fat children will become fat adults? The evidence on this point has been quite consistent over the last 15 years, but the interpretation placed on the evidence has changed. Table 9.1 sets out in summary 13 surveys, each covering more than 100 children, which have been published in the last 15 years.

Asher (1966) reviewed her experience in a clinic in Birmingham, England, and noted that 44% of the obese schoolchildren she saw had been obese before the age of five years. She found that the results of treatment of those who had been obese in infancy were particularly bad. Obesity was defined by the child's weight relative to the standard centile charts: those more than 25% above their expected weight were classified as obese. She concluded that better treatment of obesity in infancy would help to prevent intractable obesity later in life.

Eid (1970) studied the rate of weight gain of children in Sheffield, England, and related this to their weight at age 6–8 years. He concluded that rapid weight gain in the first six months of life was related to subsequent obesity, and associated this with the early introduction of cereals into the babies' feed. However, when his data are examined in the light of subsequent experience the evidence for this conclusion is not very strong. Among 138 infants who gained weight rapidly (faster than the 90th centile) in the first six months there were 28 (20.3%) who were at least 10% overweight at age 6–8 years. This is statistically a significant association, but it must be

Table 9.1 Surveys concerning the subsequent weight history of obese children

Author & date	n	Age at first survey	Age at second survey	Measure of obesity	Conclusion: does the first measurement predict the second?
Asher 1966	269	birth	1½–14 y.	wt. for ht.	44% obese children obese before 5 y.
Eid 1970	224	0–6 m.	6–8 y.	wt. for ht.	Early rapid wt. gain associated with obesity
Abraham et al 1971	717	9–13 y.	40–55 y.	wt. for ht.	Childhood weight patterns persist into adulthood
Sohar et al 1973	404	6–7 y.	13–14 y.	wt. for ht.	Relative weight determined in infancy and persists
Fisch et al 1975	1345	birth	4 & 7 y.	wt. for ht.	Most obese usually stay obese
Charney et al 1976	366	0–6 m.	20–30 y.	wt. for ht.	Infant weight correlates strongly with adult weight
Mellbin & Vuille 1973	972	0–1 y.	7 y.	wt. for ht.	Only 20% of variance explained in infancy
Poskitt & Cole 1977	203	0–1 y.	5 y.	wt. for ht. & skinfolds	Few obese babies remain obese, but obese toddlers were probably obese babies
Wilkinson et al 1977	161	0–5 y.	10 y.	wt. for ht.	43% of obese children at 10 y. had been obese at 5 y.
Sveger 1978	243	0–1 y.	2 ± ½ y.	wt. for ht.	50% of those obese at 1 y. still obese at 2 y.
Hawk & Brook 1979	621	2–15 y.	17–30 y.	skinfolds	'Moderate correlation' r = 0.5
Dine et al 1979	582	birth	5 y.	several	'Less than half variance explained in first year
Durnin & McKillop 1979	102	0–2 y.	14–16 y.	wt. for ht. & skinfolds	Very low correlation in boys, but fat girls were often fat babies

m = months, y = years, wt. = weight, ht. = height.

remembered that nearly 80% of the infants with rapid weight gain were not 10% overweight at age 6–8 years. Furthermore among the 86 infants who did not show rapid weight gain 6 (6.9%) were at least 10% overweight at age 6–8 years. These two studies therefore showed that there was a significant tendency for fat babies to be over-represented subsequently among the obese population of schoolchildren, but that by no means all fat school children had been fat babies, nor would all fat babies remain fat.

The surveys of Abraham et al (1971) in Hagerstown, U.S.A., and of Sohar et al (1973) in Tel Aviv, Israel, started with rather older children. The Hagerstown survey showed that by age 9–13 year the weight pattern for later life had been largely set. Sohar et al (1973) state 'the relative weight of both obese and non-obese subjects seems to be determined in early infancy, and tends to remain constant during childhood, adolescence and usually during adult life'. However this conclusion goes beyond their data, which concern the children's weight, as a percentage of ideal weight, at age 6–7 years and at age 13–14 years. The results are shown in Figure 9.3. At age 6–7 years there were 17 children in the heaviest group (131–150% of ideal weight) and all of these were in the same weight category at age 13–14 years. However, the less overweight children did not keep within their weight categories on follow-up, although the majority did. It can be

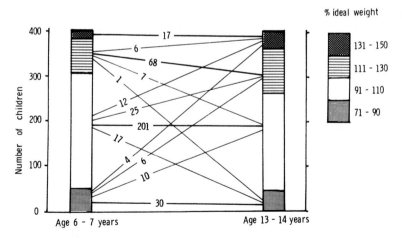

Fig. 9.3 Progression of weight, as % ideal weight for height, among 404 children studied at age 6–7 years, and again at age 13–14 years, by Sohar et al (1973). Shading indicates weight-for-height groups, and the numerals on lines indicate the number of children travelling between the weight-for-height groups joined by that line during the 7-year interval

seen from Fig 9.3 that of the 39 most-overweight children at age 13–14 years 17 came from the most-overweight group of 6–7-year-olds, but 6 came from those previously 111–130% of ideal weight, 12 from those previously 91–110%, and 4 from those previously 71–90% of ideal weight. Clearly there is a tendency for children to keep within their relative weight groups during their school days, but less than half of the most-overweight children at 13–14 years had been in the most-overweight group at 6–7 years.

The report of Fisch et al (1975) is particularly valuable, because a large series of babies were studied prospectively at birth, age 4 years and age 7 years. The ratio of weight to height was taken as a measure of obesity. The 96 children who were heaviest at birth provided a significantly larger than expected proportion of the children who were heaviest at age 4 years and 7 years (P <0.05). However when the heaviest 5% of children at age 7 years were traced back to their birthweight there were no more than might happen by chance among the heaviest at birth. Between 4 years and 7 years there was little change in ranking order for weight. Charney et al (1976) traced the adult weight of children who had been either fat, average, or thin in the first 6 months of life. Of the 32 adults who were over 120% of average weight-for-height 17 had been in the group of fattest babies, 6 had been average-weight babies, and 9 had been thin babies.

The publications reviewed so far emphasise the fact that fat children are more likely to be fat later in life than thin children. However the important question is: can the weight, or rate of weight gain, early in life be used to predict obesity later? If this is possible then children who are particularly at risk to become severely obese could be identified, and some preventive measures could be concentrated on this high-risk group. Mellbin and Vuille (1973) analysed data on 972 children in Uppsala, Sweden, to see if it was possible to predict weight for height at age 7 years from data about birth weight, birth length, monthly gain in weight during the first year, maximum monthly weight gain, or the ratio of maximum monthly gain to mean monthly gain. For both boys and girls the best single factor to predict weight-for-height at age 7 was weight gain during the first 12 months, but the correlation coefficients were low: $r = 0.056$ for girls, and $r = 0.082$ for boys. Even with the other factors added in a multiple regression analysis the data on growth in the first year could only explain 9% of the variation in weight for height at age 7 years among girls, and only 18% of the variation among boys. This is useless for effective prevention. To take one of the more promising predictive models, it might be supposed that boys who gained more than 7.5 kg in the first year would be at high risk for future obesity. There were 140 out of 465 boys who exceeded this rate of weight gain. If 10% overweight at age 7 is taken as the criterion of obesity the rapidly gaining infants were divided 33:104 between the overweight and normal weight classes at age 7, while the infants who did not have rapid weight gain in the first year were divided 27:298 between overweight and normal weight at age 7 years. If 20% overweight is taken as the criterion of obesity at age 7 years then 6:134 of the rapidly gaining infants were obese:normal, while 6:319 of the non-rapidly gaining infants were obese:normal at age 7 years. Prediction of overweight with girls was still less successful. Thus if the criteria used to predict obesity are set in such a way that one third of babies are thought to be potentially obese, this group will contain only about half of the children who eventually are found to be overweight. This is too small a catch for so wide a net.

The results of Poskett and Cole (1977) support a similar conclusion. They traced 203 children who had been surveyed at about 5 months of age, and assessed their weight-for-height and skinfold thickness. Most of the previously obese infants had returned to normal weight by the age of 5 years. Sveger (1978) also found that obese infants were no longer obese by the age of 4 years. Dine et al (1979) traced back the weight history of the heaviest 10% children at age 5 years, and found that whatever measure of obesity was used these children could not have been identified by their weight during the first year of life. Durnin and McKillop (1979) also found a low correlation between measures of fatness (weight-for-height or skinfolds) at age 0–2 years, and 14 years later.

The children studied by Hawk and Brook (1979) were rather older at the time of the first survey: between 2 and 15 years of age. When they were re-examined 15 years later the correlation between the ranking of the skinfold measurements at first and second examination was 0.56 for male and 0.45 for female subjects. This is a rather better level of prediction than that achieved from measurements in the first year of life, but still not very impressive. Better correlations were obtained by Zack et al (1979) from the data of the U.S. Health Examination Surveys of 2,177 children at age 6–11 years and again at age 12–17 years. Of the children who were in the 20% most obese at the time of the first survey about 70% were in the correspondingly obese group at the time of the second survey, and about 20% were in the next-most-obese category.

Thus, while it is true that obese and lean adults do not always remain obese and lean (Garn and Cole 1980), and it is also true that extremely obese adults were probably obese as children (Rimm and Rimm 1976), it is not true that obesity in the first year of life is highly correlated with obesity thereafter. During the first two or three years of life children change weight categories quite freely, but by the age of 6 years those who are likely to be obese have usually declared themselves (see Fig 9.3) although there is still considerable mobility in the moderately overweight category. This is not to say that a child who reaches the age of 6 years at normal weight has escaped the perils of obesity: in the series of obese 10-year-olds reviewed by Wilkinson et al (1977) over half had not been obese at age 5 years.

TREATMENT OF OBESITY IN CHILDHOOD

Exactly the same principles of energy balance apply to the treatment of obesity in children or adults: the child became obese because it took in more energy than it required for normal growth and development, and the cure lies in reducing energy intake slightly below requirements so the excess fat is used up. However there are special factors in the management of obese children, of which the most important is that instead of there being a two-party relationship between the obese adult patient and the therapist there is a triangular relationship between the obese child, its parent and the therapist. In the case of young children the problem is to convince the mother that the suggested line of treatment is in the interests of the child, but with adolescent children the situation is very complex. There is no sight more discouraging to a doctor in an obesity clinic than the entry of a thin, anxious, fussy mother followed by her scowling obese adolescent daughter. Probably there is no period of life at which treatment for obesity is so unsuccessful as between the age of 12 and 16 years. Before that age the child may comply with dietary regulations imposed by the parents and school, after that age the obese young adult may take responsibility for dietary control, but between those ages the adolescent impulse to rebel against authority leaves little scope for dietary supervision unless the child can somehow be persuaded that weight loss is a problem for him or her to tackle, and that any credit for success will belong to the child, and not to the parent.

The other special factor in management of obesity in children is that the child has more stringent nutrient requirements than an adult if normal growth and development is to proceed.

Nutrient requirements of children

The recommended daily amounts of food energy and nutrients for groups of children is set out in Table 9.2. (Department of Health and Social Security 1979). The notable features of the nutrient requirements of children, compared with those of adults, are that they require relatively more energy, protein and calcium to support normal growth.

Table 9.2 Nutrient requirements of children (data from DHSS report 1979)

Age yrs	Energy kcal	MJ	Protein g	Thiamin mg	Riboflavin mg	Nicotinic acid mg	Total folate µg	Ascorbic acid mg	Vitamin A µg	Vitamin D µg	Calcium mg	Iron mg
BOYS												
1	1200	5.0	30	0.5	0.6	7	100	20	300	10	600	7
2	1400	5.8	35	0.6	0.7	8	100	20	300	10	600	7
3–4	1560	6.5	39	0.6	0.8	9	100	20	300	10	600	8
5–6	1740	7.3	43	0.7	0.9	10	200	20	300		600	10
7–8	1980	8.3	49	0.8	1.0	11	200	20	400		600	10
9–11	2280	9.5	57	0.9	1.2	14	200	25	575		600	12
12–14	2640	11.0	66	1.1	1.4	16	300	25	725		700	12
15–17	2880	12.0	72	1.2	1.7	19	300	30	750		600	12
GIRLS												
1	1100	4.5	27	0.4	0.6	7	100	20	300	10	600	7
2	1300	5.5	32	0.5	0.7	8	100	20	300	10	600	7
3–4	1500	6.3	37	0.6	0.8	9	100	20	300	10	600	8
5–6	1680	7.0	42	0.7	0.9	10	200	20	300		600	10
7–8	1900	8.0	47	0.8	1.0	11	200	20	400		600	10
9–11	2050	8.5	51	0.8	1.2	14	300	25	575		600	12
12–14	2150	9.0	53	0.9	1.4	16	300	25	725		700	12
15–17	2150	9.0	53	0.9	1.7	19	300	30	750		600	12

The recommended intakes for children deserve to be treated with rather more respect than those for adults (see page 99) because there have been more metabolic balance studies done on children than adults, and in children there are criteria of growth to indicate dietary inadequacy, but there are no such indices in the assessment of adult nutrition.

Fortunately it is never necessary, or desirable, to achieve rapid weight loss in children, so moderate dietary restriction is all that is necessary. The problems which arise with very-low energy diets with adults can therefore be avoided. However it is important to realise that energy requirements among children show just as large a range of variation between individuals as is found among adults (Widdowson 1962). The objective is to slow down the child's rate of weight increase so that with the natural increase in height he or she achieves normal proportions. This is a very long-term and unspectacular objective, and many parents and children do not have the patience to pursue it.

Motivation to control weight

Chapter 2 of this book concerns the cost:benefit ratio for overweight adults who are considering how hard they should try to lose weight. For children it is difficult to make a case that it is in their interests to lose weight, not because there is little advantage in controlling obesity in childhood, but because these advantages are so remote in time that they have little impact on the child. Even among adolescents the motivation to lose weight is often mainly based on hopes of social benefit, which may or may not be realised. Obesity causes very little physical disability in children: the fat child will often find a niche, such as goal-keeper, in which he performs well even in games. At swimming their natural buoyancy actually helps fat children.

The main disability affecting the obese child at school is the disapproval of other pupils. DeJong (1980) showed that high school girls aged 14 to 18 years held quite strong prejudices against obese schoolfellows. Girls were asked to participate in a study about 'first impressions' and were given a data sheet containing information about another girl who was said to have been a participant in a previous course. In fact fictitious data sheets were used, so the replies to the questionnaires indicated the girls' opinion of a schoolfellow who was obese or normal in build, and for each build the data sheets indicated that the girl either had some thyroid trouble or was quite healthy. The obese girl who was perfectly healthy was least liked: if she had the excuse of thyroid trouble for her obesity the rating was somewhat better. In a second experiment an obese girl who was said to be losing weight was more acceptable than one who seemed not to mind about her obesity. These results indicate that children blame obese children for their obesity, which they regard as a sign of greed, sloth, and similar disagreeable characteristics. DeJong concludes that children should be educated to be more tolerant of obesity in their fellows, since the aetiology of obesity is complex, and not necessarily the fault of the obese child.

This conclusion is very reasonable, but it does nothing to solve the problem of how to get the obese child to lose weight. It is clearly bad to reinforce the social stigma of obesity by suggesting that it is the fault of the child that he or she is fat, but if we go to the other extreme and say that it is an Act of God about which nothing can be done this cuts out any hope of successful treatment. Such an attitude is anyway false: something can be done. The delicate problem is to get the child to try to tackle the obesity without being unduly critical. It is easier to establish rapport with the child if it turns out that he or she is better-than-average (at least in his or her estimation) at something — say memorising poetry, or singing in tune, or playing an instrument. The child will usually concede that it is lucky for him or her to have this talent, and unlucky for others to have to invest greater effort to achieve the same result in the sphere at which this talent applies. It may then seem less unjust that in another sphere, that of maintaining a normal weight, the obese child has to invest greater effort than others to achieve the same result.

Even if the child accepts this rather sophisticated argument it is by no means certain that the parents will be satisfied with it. They either think that the child's food intake is perfectly normal, so the obesity must be caused by a glandular abnormality which it is the duty of the doctor to diagnose, or else that the child must be secretly gorging. The problem of investigating the child to satisfy the parents has been discussed on page 181. The problem of parents who take a punitive view of their fat children is less easily dealt with. If possible they should be persuaded that the best policy is to concentrate on what is best for the child in the future, and to forget any arguments about the cause of the obesity. The child is too fat because he or she has eaten slightly more than was required, and it is fruitless to speculate if that was because food intake was a bit higher than average, or requirements a bit lower than average, since all this is in the past and cannot now be determined. The most useful thing which the parents can now do is to make it as easy as possible for the child to follow the appropriate dietary advice, and to give it every encouragement with whatever it achieves in the way of controlling its weight.

Results of treatment of obese children

Generally the results of published series, where weight change has been measured over several years, are not encouraging (Lloyd et al 1961). In a more recent review Coates and Thorensen (1978) say 'Treatment approaches used to date are generally impotent'. Brownwell and Stunkard (1978b) are rather more optimistic about the results of behavioural treatment of obesity in children. However treatment programmes which involve monetary deposits, refundable in part for attendance, the completion of charts and graphs, and for weight loss, are practicable only for middle-class families with cooperative parents. This limitation of behaviour therapy for adults has been pointed out by Weisenberg and Frey (1974). Furthermore there is a risk that, if the child is encouraged to indulge in excessive introspection about the circumstances in which it eats, the good which is achieved by weight loss will be offset by damage to the normal psychological development of the child.

A programme for weight control which is applicable to children of any social class or background is described by Choksi et al (1980). They accepted obese children aged 9–16 years at a district hospital in Chicago: none was rejected on the basis of poor motivation or financial reasons. The programme consisted of weekly group sessions for discussion, exercise and nutrition education. Each week a small reward was made according to a points system based on attendance, maintenance of a diet record, and weight loss: this was financed from a contribution of H5.00 per month from participating parents, which was the only cost to the patient of attendance in the programme. There were 33 girls and 6 boys in the treatment group. Of these only 17 lost more than 5 lb (2 kg) during the study period of 15 months, but 35 showed a slowing of weight gain relative to height gain, so they came closer to the normal weight-for-height.

This slowing in the rate of weight gain is a reasonable objective in the treatment of obese children. It is probably more useful to the child in the long term to proceed fairly gradually in controlling weight, which will be a problem for many years. The evidence suggests that inpatient treatment of obese children with substantial weight reduction does not confer lasting benefit (Lloyd et al 1961).

10

Summary and guidelines on the treatment of obesity

Obesity is one of the most important health hazards in affluent countries. The risks to health and disabilities of overweight people are reduced by weight loss. The greatest risk to health, and hence the greatest potential benefit from weight loss, is among young adults who are severely overweight, so this group deserve priority in treatment for obesity.

Ideally the obese person should take a diet which provides 500–1000 kcal (2–4 MJ) less than energy requirements, but which provides adequate amounts of all nutrients other than energy. The energy deficit will be met by using some of the excess stored fat, and in the long term this loss of adipose tissue will be reflected by an average rate of weight loss of 0.5–1 kg (1–2 lb) per week. Initially higher rates of weight loss will probably be observed, for reasons explained in Chapter 3.

Larger energy deficits can be achieved — for example by total starvation — and will be associated with higher rates of weight loss. However this is not good for the obese persons, since high rates of weight loss are associated with excessive loss of lean tissue, not fat. If lean tissue is lost the resting metabolic rate decreases, and it becomes even more difficult for the patient to maintain weight loss. Slow rates of weight loss, associated with smaller energy deficits, are unsatisfactory to any but the slightly overweight.

Since people differ in lifestyle and energy requirements reducing diets need to be adjusted to the needs of individual patients. Ideally dietary counselling should be done by a trained dietitian. For those without professional dietetic help the outline of a general-purpose reducing diet is given in Appendix 1 of this book. The nutrients associated with food groups, and the protein and energy content of 100 g portions of some common foods, are listed in Appendix 2. If patients make their own selection of foods within a certain daily energy limit — say 1000 kcal (4 MJ) — they may choose a diet with inadequate protein.

There is no food item — salads, citrus fruits, bran — which is especially helpful in promoting satiety or in mobilising fat. Generally the capacity of food to reduce hunger is roughly in proportion to the energy content of the food with the exception of alcohol, which is a source of energy but does not proportionately reduce hunger. It is not essential that a reducing diet should be taken at fixed mealtimes, but the ratio of fat loss to lean tissue loss is more favourable if a diet with a fairly high protein content is taken in frequent meals, than if an isoenergetic diet with less protein is taken as a single meal (see page 130). There is no advantage in restricting the amount of water taken with a reducing diet. People who are unwilling to count calories may prefer 'no counting' or 'low carbohydrate' diets (pp. 163–165). Provided that these diets result in an equivalent reduction in energy intake they are as satisfactory as calorie-counted diets.

People on reducing diets should be encouraged to take exercise, since this promotes fitness. However exercise alone is usually ineffective in causing significant weight loss. There is no evidence that exercise reduces appetite.

Anorectic drugs of the phenylethylamine group are effective in reducing hunger, but work better when given intermittently than continuously. Fenfluramine must not be given intermittently. Controlled trials show that much of the effectiveness of drug treatment for weight reduction is a placebo effect: it encourages the patient to try harder with the diet. Anorectic drugs should not be given in short courses to 'start patients off' on a reducing diet: if they are used at all it should probably be for long periods in selected patients. Surveys indicate that patients who have experience of dieting with or without drugs usually prefer in the long run to manage without drugs.

There is currently great interest in drugs which increase the metabolic rate, and hence cause a greater energy deficit for a given diet. Thyroid hormones have been extensively used for this purpose, and do cause greater weight loss, but the extra weight loss is mostly lean tissue, so this is not to the advantage of the patient. Probably other thermogenic drugs will be promoted, but such drugs must always carry some risk, since any increase in the resting metabolic rate of an obese patient necessarily reduces exercise tolerance.

Drugs which reduce the absorption of energy from the gut are being tested as a treatment for obesity. Any dietary energy which becomes unavailable to the patient as a result of this treatment will become available to his colonic bacteria. It is predictable that even a small decrease in energy absorbed from the gut will support a large increase in fermentation and gas production in the large bowel, and this effect will limit the usefulness of this line of treatment.

Over the last 10 years behaviour therapy for obesity, pioneered by Stuart, has been adapted and applied in many weight-control programmes. It was hoped that obese people would learn new 'normal' eating patterns, and hence achieve permanent weight loss. Stuart's original results have not been replicated on a wide scale, and maintenance of weight loss, although better than that achieved after a finite period of drug treatment, has not been as good as the early follow-up studies suggested. It is not yet clear how the principles of behaviour modification can most effectively be applied in the large-scale management of obesity. Social pressures may cause some women to attempt to maintain an unnaturally low body weight: this gives rise to problems with unnecessary dieting and 'compulsive eating' which are discussed in Chapter 7.

Obesity in pregnancy presents the obstetrician with a dilemma. If the mother's diet is too severely restricted the growth of the baby may be impaired, while if no attempt is made to deal with the mother's obesity while she is susceptible to dietary advice a valuable opportunity will be lost. A satisfactory compromise is to attempt to limit the weight gain of obese women during pregnancy to about half the normal amount: this policy is in the best interests of both the mother and her baby.

The hypothesis of Hirsch, that the number of fat cells — possibly determined by feeding in infancy — determines subsequent obesity, is not generally accepted today. The technical difficulties associated with this theory are discussed on page 182. Although very fat babies tend to become fat adults there is considerable change in adiposity-ranking among children during infancy and early childhood. It is prudent to try to prevent an infant from becoming obese, but there is no good evidence of a critical period of life at which future obesity is determined.

From the outline of treatment methods given above it is evident that the problem in treating obesity does not arise from any lack of effective therapeutic regimens. Once an obese person is an inpatient in a well-run metabolic ward it is possible — given enough time — to achieve virtually any desired reduction in adipose tissue without excessive loss of lean tissue. There are two main difficulties in putting therapeutic principles into practice with outpatients. First, it is necessary for the person who wants to lose weight to spend enough time with a well-informed therapist to learn how this can be achieved. For some people it is enough to be given a diet sheet: these people would anyway obtain the information they need from magazines and would not go to the general practitioner. For many others a diet sheet is not enough: they require hours of advice, encouragement, and more advice when things go wrong. The second problem concerns the doctor-patient relationship, to which I will return later.

The solution to the problem of therapist-time must be some form of group treatment. One-to-one dietary counselling involves inefficient use of the time both of the patient and of the doctor or dietitian. The patient spends time unprofitably in the waiting-room, conscious that dietary advice ranks low in the list of priorities of most general practitioners. The doctor has inadequate time (and often inadequate training and inclination also) to give this advice in competition with other calls on his services. On the other hand the slimming group of about 15–20 people with similar interests is a very efficient educational system. In a ten-week course, with two-hour sessions every week, each course member gets 20 hours of relevant instruction, and the opportunity to see the results obtained within the group, at a cost of only 20 hours of therapist time. It is practicable to use teaching aids such as films, and such courses can be self-financing at little cost to the course-member (Seddon et al 1981).

Of course a dietitian-led slimming group is not the answer to the whole problem of obesity, but it is a very effective first step. Perhaps half the members will achieve a satisfactory rate of weight loss, and of the remainder some will not be very serious about losing weight anyway. It is on the small proportion of members who really want and need to lose weight, but who fail to do so in the group, that the hospital-based obesity clinic should most profitably concentrate. If referrals to the hospital clinic were filtered through a well-run slimming club the expensive hospital facilities would be used to greater effect.

The possible investigations and lines of treatment available in hospital are described in the earlier part of this book. Often investigation of a severely obese (grade III) patient will reveal no metabolic abnormality — the difficulty is that the patient cannot keep to a restricted diet for long enough to achieve the weight loss on which his or her future health depends. For reasons set out in Chap. 4, pp. 67–76, the most effective line of treatment in such a situation is step-wise approach. First try a milk diet. If that fails go on to to jaw wiring, with a waist cord to control weight gain when the wires are removed, or if that fails a gastric reduction procedure.

It is at this point that the second problem arises, that of the doctor-patient relationship. This topic has recently come under the scrutiny of the 1980 Reith Lecturer whose final talk concerned consumerism in the doctor-patient relationship

'In the practice of medicine the consumer is the patient. His interests, which consumerism would seek to assert, are those of self-determination and the power to participate responsibly in decisions made about his life. The challenge to that power comes from the doctor, who, in the exercise of his professional role, threatens to infantilise the patient, to undermine his power of self-determination, to act in a paternalistic manner'. (Kennedy 1980).

Here, then, is a trap. If the doctor tries to force the patient to diet he is acting against the patient's interest in self-determination. However, if he says it is entirely up to the patient to diet or not as he pleases, he is also acting against the patient's interests, since it is a mockery to pretend that the patient could diet unaided.

The way out of this dilemma concerns informed consent. As Kennedy (1980) puts it: 'Informed consent flies the flag of self-determination against the otherwise ever-present paternalism of the doctor'. Before a doctor can ethically help a severely obese patient it is necessary that both parties understand what options are available, and the probable advantages and disadvantages associated with each line of treatment, or non-treatment. This book is an attempt to set out this information for the people who need it.

Appendix 1
Weight-reducing diet

The diet below is used by the Dietetic Department, Harrow Health District. The number of slices of bread per day is adjusted to provide the required energy content. With 2 large slices of bread (3 oz, or 80 g) or equivalent in exchanges, this diet provides about 1000 kcal (4 MJ) per day.

Suggested meal pattern
Use milk from your allowance for tea, coffee and cereal.

Early morning	Tea or coffee — no sugar.
Breakfast	Grapefruit or juice or fruit from allowance. Egg or small portion of bacon, ham or fish or cheese if desired. Tomatoes or mushrooms if desired (NO FAT) ....slices of bread with butter or margarine from allowance OR........cereal. Tea or coffee — no sugar.
Mid morning	Tea or coffee — no sugar. or low calorie squash or Bovril or Oxo.
Mid day or evening	Clear Soup. Lean meat, fish, cheese, egg or liver. Salad or green vegetable as desired or root vegetable. ....slices bread OR........potatoes. Fruit from allowance.
Mid afternoon	Tea or coffee — no sugar. or low calorie drink, e.g. squash, or Bovril, Oxo.
Evening or mid day	Clear soup. Lean meat, fish, cheese, egg or liver. Salad or green vegetables. ....slices bread OR........potatoes. Fruit from allowance.
Bedtime	Tea or coffee OR rest of milk from allowance. OR low calorie squash or Bovril or Oxo.

Food portion guide

Lean meat	50 g (2 oz) per cooked portion. This includes beef, lamb, pork, poultry, ham, bacon, liver. BUT you must not fry or use thickened gravies.
Fish	100 g (4 oz) per cooked portion. You may take all kinds of fish. BUT no fried fish or thickened sauces. Drain the oil off tinned fish.
Cheese	25 g (1 oz) per portion of hard cheese, e.g. Cheddar, 100 g (4 oz) per portion cottage cheese. Avoid cream cheese, cheese spread.

Egg	Boiled or poached only. 1 or 2 eggs per portion.
Milk	Keep to 250 ml (½ pint) a day or 500 ml (1 pint) skimmed milk or 4 tbls skimmed milk powder. Alternatively 150 ml (¼ pint) milk + carton plain unsweetened yoghurt.
Fruit	3 helpings. These can be fresh, frozen, cooked, or tinned in water and includes oranges, apples, pears, peaches, plums, strawberries, blackberries, etc. If sweetening is necessary, use saccharin. In cooking, it should be added at the end just before serving, otherwise a bitter taste will develop. A glass of unsweetened pineapple, orange, tomato or grapefruit juice counts as a helping of fruit.
Root & pulse vegetables	Not more than one tablespoon per day of carrots, parsnips, beetroot, peas, broad beans, sweetcorn, turnips.
Butter or Margarine	Not more than 10 g (¹/₃ oz) per day (or 20 g – ²/₃ oz low fat spread). 75 g (3 oz) should last you a week.
Bread	. . . . .slices from large medium cut loaf.
Exchanges	1 slice large loaf (40 g) can be exchanged for the following: 2 small thin cut slices bread 75 g boiled rice — 2 heaped tablespoons 2 Potatoes, size of an egg 75 g boiled spaghetti (15 strands raw) 25 g unsweetened breakfast cereal — 5 tablespoons, preferably wholewheat 3 crispbread 2 Pieces of fruit 2 semi-sweet biscuits or cream crackers

You may eat the following foods freely

Green vegetables	Cabbage, greens, sprouts, cauliflower, green beans, spinach, brocolli, marrow, mushrooms, onions, aubergines
Salads	Lettuce, tomato, cucumber, radishes, celery, spring onions, chicory, cress
Soups	Clear Soups, stock cubes, Bovril, Marmite, Oxo.
Pickles	Pickles in vinegar, e.g. gherkins, Worcester sauce, salt, mustard, pepper, herbs and spices.
Other	Tea, coffee, sodawater, low calorie squashes, sugar-free fizzy drinks, natural P.L.J. etc., saccharin tablet or liquid.

Foods to avoid

Sugary foods	Sugar, glucose, jam, honey, marmalade, syrup, treacle. Chocolates, peppermints and confectionery Ice cream, ice lollies, jellies, fruit yoghurts, instant desserts and mousses.
Fatty foods	Fried foods, dripping, oil, lard, cream, tinned milk, salad cream, mayonnaise and salad dressing.
Drinks	Sweet fruit Squashes, soft drinks, sweetened fizzy drinks, e.g. Lucozade and lemonade. Cocoa and malted milk drinks.
Alcohol	Beer, stout, ale, cider, spirits, wine and sherry.
Cereals	Sugar-coated breakfast cereals, muesli, semolina, sago, tapioca, rice in puddings, cakes, pastry, pies, scones, tinned spaghetti.
Fruit	Tinned fruit in syrup or sorbitol, bananas, grapes, nuts, dried fruit.

Proprietary   Slimming foods and diabetic foods (except squashes), powdered
foods   sweeteners.

Vegetables   Butter beans, baked beans, barley, lentils, crisps.

It is advisable to eat foods rich in iron such as liver, kidney and corned beef regularly.

Appendix 2
Energy and protein content of common foods

The energy and protein content of some common foods are listed in the following sequence:

Meat and meat products
Eggs
Fish
Milk and cream
Cheese
Bread
Cereals, cakes and biscuits
Fats and oils
Sugar and preserves
Vegetables
Fruit and nuts
Beverages and soft drinks.

Values have been taken from Paul and Southgate (1978) and refer to 100 g portions of food as normally eaten, (eg. meat, cooked, without bone).

Estimates of average consumption of each food group are derived from the National Food Survey for 1978.

Energy value of common foods, and their chief nutritional significance

Meat and meat products
Source of about 16% of energy and 35% of protein intake by average household. Average consumption 140 g/day. Important source of Fe, P and B vitamins, but expensive.

	Energy		Protein
	kcal	MJ	g
Bacon, fried, average	480	1.9	24
grilled, average	410	1.7	25
Beef, sirloin, roast	280	1.2	24
Lamb, roast	410	1.7	19
Pork, chops, grilled	330	1.4	28
Veal, fillet, roast	230	1.0	32
Chicken, roast	210	0.9	23
Duck, roast	340	1.4	20

	Energy		Protein
	kcal	MJ	g
Turkey, roast	170	0.7	28
Rabbit, stewed	180	0.7	27
Kidney, ox, stewed	170	0.7	26
Liver, calf, fried	250	1.0	27
Tongue, ox, boiled	290	1.2	19
Beef, corned	210	0.9	27
Sausages, pork, fried	320	1.3	14
pork, grilled	320	1.3	14

Eggs
Source of about 2% of energy and 5% of protein intake by average household. High cholesterol content.

	Energy		Protein
	kcal	MJ	g
Eggs, boiled	150	0.6	12
fried	230	1.0	14
scrambled	250	1.0	11

Fish
Source of about 1% of energy and 5% of protein intake by average household. Average consumption 17 g/day. Fatty fishes have higher energy content. Fish oils rich in vitamins A and D. Seafood has high iodine content.

	Energy		Protein
	kcal	MJ	g
Cod, grilled	90	0.4	21
fried in batter	200	0.8	20
Haddock, fried	170	0.7	21
Lemon sole, fried	220	0.9	16
Mackerel, fried	190	0.8	22
Salmon, steamed	200	0.8	20
smoked	140	0.6	25
Lobster, boiled	120	0.5	22
Scampi, fried	320	1.3	12

Milk and cream
Source of about 15% of energy and 17% of protein intake of average household. Average consumption 375 g/day. Sole food for infants: important source of many nutrients, especially Ca and P, but not of Fe or vitamins C or D.

	Energy		Protein
	kcal	MG	g
Milk, cows', fresh, whole	65	0.3	3.3
fresh, skimmed	33	0.14	3 4
Cream, single	210	0.9	2.4
double	450	1.8	1.5

Cheese
Source of about 2% of energy and 7% of protein intake of average household. Average consumption 17 g/day. Important source of Ca, vitamin A and riboflavin.

	Energy		Protein
	kcal	MJ	g
Camembert	300	1.2	23
Cheddar	400	1.7	26

	Energy kcal	MJ	Protein g
Danish blue	350	1.5	23
Stilton	460	1.9	26
Cottage cheese	100	0.4	14

Bread

Source of about 15% of energy and 16% of protein intake of average households. Average consumption 140 g/day. Nutrient content affected by milling of grain: wholemeal flour (100% extraction) contains more fibre than white flour (70% extraction). Wheat bran contains B vitamins, Ca, Fe and Zn, but also phytate which inhibits absorption of these minerals.

	Energy kcal	MJ	Protein g
Bread, wholemeal	220	0.9	8.8
white	230	1.0	7.8
malt	248	1.1	8.3
Rolls, crusty	290	1.2	11.6

Cereals, cakes, biscuits

Source of about 12% of energy and 6% of protein intake of average household. Average consumption 80 g/day. Nutritional significance similar to that of bread.

	Energy kcal	MJ	Protein g
Bran, wheat	210	0.9	14
Oatmeal, raw	400	1.7	12
Spaghetti, boiled	120	0.5	4.2
Cornflakes	370	1.6	8.6
Cream crackers	440	1.9	9.5
Crispbread, rye	320	1.4	9.4
Biscuit, digestive, plain	470	2.0	9.8
chocolate	490	2.1	6.8
shortbread	500	2.1	6.2
Cake, fruit, rich	330	1.4	3.7
gingerbread	370	1.6	6.1
sponge, without fat	300	1.3	10.0
Doughnuts	350	1.5	6.0
Pastry, shortcrust	530	2.2	6.9
Pancakes	310	1.3	6.1
Treacle tart	370	1.6	3.8

Fats and oils

Provides 15% of energy intake, and negligible protein. Vitamin content of butter is variable: margarine is fortified with vitamin A and D. Average consumption 40 g/day.

	Energy kcal	MJ	Protein g
Butter, margarine	740	3.0	—
Vegetable oil, lard, dripping	900	3.7	—

Sugar and preserves
Source of about 10% of energy intake of average household. Negligible contribution to
nutrition otherwise. Average consumption about 60 g/day.

	Energy		Protein
	kcal	MJ	g
Sugar, white or Demerara	400	1.7	—
Syrup, golden	300	1.3	—
Honey, comb	280	1.2	—
Jam, fruit with edible seeds	260	1.1	0.6
Marmalade	260	1.1	—
Chocolate, milk	530	2.2	8.4
plain	520	2.2	4.7
Toffee	430	1.8	2.1

Vegetables
Source of about 7% of energy intake and 8% of protein intake of average household.
Potato (180 g/day) accounts for the major part of vegetable consumption (340 g/day)
and for an even higher proportion of nutrient intake from this group. Food values are
affected by freshness of vegetables, processing and cooking.

	Energy		Protein
	kcal	MJ	g
Potatoes, boiled	80	0.34	1.4
baked, with skin	85	0.36	2.1
roast	160	0.66	2.8
chips	250	1.06	3.8
crisps	530	2.22	6.3
Beans, runner, boiled	20	0.08	1.9
broad, boiled	50	0.2	4.1
Beetroot, boiled	40	0.2	1.8
Brussels sprouts, boiled	20	0.08	2.8
Cabbage, white, raw	20	0.09	1.9
Carrots, boiled	20	0.08	0.6
Celery, raw	8	0.04	0.9
Lettuce, raw	10	0.05	1.0
Mushrooms, raw	10	0.5	1.8
fried	210	0.9	2.2
Mustard and cress, raw	10	0.05	1.6
Onions, boiled	10	0.5	0.6
fried	350	1.4	1.8
Parsnips, boiled	60	0.2	1.3
Peas, fresh, boiled	50	220	5.0
Tomatoes, raw	10	0.06	0.9
fried	70	0.3	1.0

Fruit and nuts
Source of about 2% of energy intake and 1% of protein intake of average household.
Average consumption 90 g/day. Important source of vitamin C, especially from raw and
citrus fruit. Generally low energy concentration, since weight is mostly water and
cellulose.

	Energy		Protein
	kcal	MJ	g
Apples, eating, raw	50	0.2	0.3
Avocado pear	220	0.9	4.2
Banana, raw	80	0.3	1.1

	Energy		Protein
	kcal	MJ	g
Cherries, raw	50	0.2	0.6
Damson, raw	40	0.2	0.5
Dates, dried	250	1.1	2.0
Gooseberries, raw	20	0.07	1.1
stewed with sugar	50	0.2	0.9
Grapes, raw	60	0.3	0.6
Grapefruit, raw	50	0.2	0.8
Melon, Honeydew, raw	20	0.1	0.6
Oranges, raw	40	0.2	0.8
Peaches, raw	40	0.2	0.6
Pears, raw	40	0.2	0.3
Raspberries, raw	30	0.1	0.9
Strawberries, raw	30	0.1	0.6
Sultanas, dried	250	1.1	1.8
Almonds	560	2.4	16.9
Coconut, fresh	350	1.4	3.2
Peanuts, roasted and salted	570	2.4	24.3
Walnuts	530	2.2	10.6

Beverages
Infusions of coffee and tea (without added milk or sugar) have negligible nutritional value except as vehicles for water. They contain the stimulant caffeine.

Soft drinks and alcoholic beverages
Contribution to average energy intake not known, since they are often consumed outside the home and are not monitored in the National Food Survey. Beer, spirits and wines provided about 160 kcal (0.7 MJ) per head of population per day in 1975. Soft drinks may contribute significant energy to the diet, especially for people on reducing diets.

	Energy		Protein
	kcal	MJ	g
Coca-cola	40	0.2	—
Grapefruit juice, sweetened	40	0.2	—
Lucozade	70	0.3	—
Orange juice, unsweetened	30	0.1	—
sweetened	50	0.2	—
Tomato juice, canned	20	0.07	0.7
Beer (most types)	30	0.15	—
strong ale	70	0.3	—
Cider, sweet or dry	40	0.16	—
vintage	100	0.4	—
Wine, dry	70	0.3	—
sweet	90	0.4	—
Port	160	0.6	—
Sherry	120	0.5	—
Spirits, 70% proof	220	0.9	—

References

Abraham, S., Collins, G. & Nordseik, M. (1971) Relationship of childhood weight status to morbidity in adults. *Health Services and Mental Health Administration Health Reports*, **86**, 273–284.

Abraham, S. & Johnson, C. L. (1980) Prevalence of severe obesity in adults in the United States. *American Journal of Clinical Nutrition*, **33**, 364–369.

Abramson, E. E. (1977) Behavioural approaches to weight control: an updated review. *Behaviour Research and Therapy*, **15**, 355–364.

Acheson, K. J., Campbell, I. T., Edholm, O. G., Miller, D. S. & Stock, M. J. (1980a) The measurement of food and energy intake in man — an evaluation of some techniques. *American Journal of Clinical Nutrition*, **33**, 1147–1154.

Acheson, K. J., Campbell, I. T., Edholm, O. G., Miller, D. S. & Stock, M. J. (1980b) The measurement of daily energy expenditure — an evaluation of some techniques. *American Journal of Clinical Nutrition*, **33**, 1155–1164.

Addis, T., Poo, L. J. & Lew, W. (1936) Protein loss from the liver during a two-day fast. *Journal of Biological Chemistry*, **115**, 117–118.

Adolph, E. F. (1947) Urges to eat and drink in rats. *American Journal of Physiology*, **151**, 110–125.

Aja, J. H. (1977) Brief group treatment of obesity through ancillary self-hypnosis. *American Journal of Clinical Hypnosis*, **19**, 231–234.

Allan, M. (1974) *The joy of slimming*, London, Wolfe Publishing.

Allen, D. W. & Quigley, B. M. (1977) The role of physical activity in the control of obesity. *Medical Journal of Australia*, **2**, 434–438.

Allon, N. (1975 The stigma of overweight in everyday life. In *Obesity in Perspective*, ed. Bray, G. pp 83–102. U.S. Government Printing Office, Washington.

Andersen, T., Juhl, E. & Quaade, F. (1980) Jejunoileal bypass for obesity — what can we learn from a literature study? *American Journal of Clinical Nutrition 33*, 440–445.

Andres, R. (1980) Effect of obesity on total mortality. *International Journal of Obesity*, **4**, 381–386.

Anonymous (1978) Statement by the American Dietetic Association on diet protein products. *Journal of the American Dietetic Association*, **73**, 547–548.

Apfelbaum, M. (1976) The effects of very restrictive high protein diets. *Clinics in Endocrinology and Metabolism*, **5**, 417–430.

Apfelbaum, M., Bost-Sarron, J., Brigant, L. & Dupin, H. (1967) La composition du poids perdu au cours de la diete hydrique. *Gastroenterologia*, **108**, 121–134.

Ashby, W. A. & Wilson, G. T. (1977) Behaviour therapy for obesity: Booster sessions and long term maintenance of weight loss. *Behaviour Research and Therapy*, **15**, 451–463.

Asher, P. (1966) Fat babies and fat children. The prognosis for obesity in the very young. *Archives of Disease in Childhood*, **41**, 672–673.

Ashwell, M. A. (1973) A survey investigating patients' views on doctors' treatment of obesity. *Practitioner*, **211**, 653–658.

Ashwell, M. (1978a) The 'fat cell pool' concept. *International Journal of Obesity*, **2**, 69–72.

Ashwell, M. (1978b) Commercial weight loss groups. In: *Recent Advances in Obesity Research: 2*, ed. Bray, G. pp. 266–276. London, Newman Publishing.

Ashwell, M. A. (1979) How can research into fat cells and fat distribution help the treatment of obesity? *International Journal of Obesity*, **3**, 188–189.

Ashwell, M. A. & Etchell, L. (1974) Attitude of the individual to his own body weight. *British Journal of Preventive and Social Medicine*, **28**, 127–132.

Ashwell, M. A. & Garrow, J. S. (1975) A survey of three slimming and weight control organisations in the U.K. *Nutrition* (London) **29**, 347–356.

Ashwork, A. & Wolff, H. S. (1969) A simple method for measuring calorie expenditure during sleep. *Pflugers Archives: European Journal of Physiology*, **306**, 191–194.

Astwood, E. B. (1962) The heritage of corpulence. *Endocrinology*, **71**, 337–341.

Atkinson, R. L., Greenway, F. L., Bray, G. A., Dahms, W. T., Molitch, M. E., Hamilton, K. & Rodin, J. (1977) Treatment of obesity: comparison of physician and non-physician therapists using placebo and anorectic drugs in a double-blind trial. *International Journal of Obesity*, **1**, 113–120.

Atwater, W. O. & Benedict, F. G. (1899) Experiments on the metabolism of matter and energy in the human body. *Bulletin U.S. Department of Agriculture* **69**.

Atwater, W. O. & Benedict, F. G. (1905) A respiration calorimeter with appliances for the direct determination of oxygen. *Carnegie Institution of Washington*, Publication **42**.

Azizi, F. (1978) The effect of dietary composition on fasting-induced changes in serum thyroid hormones and thyrotropin. *Metabolism*, **27**, 935–942.

Bae, J., Ting, E. Y. & Gioffrida, J. G. (1976) The effect of changes in the body position of obese patients on pulmonary volume and ventilatory function. *Bulletin of the New York Academy of Medicine*, **52**, 830–837.

Baird, I. McL., Parsons, R. L. & Howard, A. N. (1974) Clinical and metabolic studies of chemically defined diets in the management of obesity. *Metabolism*, **23**, 645–657.

Baird, J. D. (1973) The role of obesity in the development of clinical diabetes. In *Anorexia and obesity*, ed. Robertson, R. F. pp. 83–99. Royal College of Physicians Publication 42, Edinburgh.

Bateson, M. (1979) Dietary advice and obesity. *British Medical Journal*, **ii**, 1585.

Beazley, J. M. & Swinhoe, J. R. (1979) Body weight in parous women: is there any alteration between successive pregnancies? *Acta Obstetrica et Gynecologica Scandinavica*, **58**, 45–47.

Behnke, A. R., Feen, B. G. & Welham, W. C. (1942) The specific gravity of healthy men: Body weight + volume as an index of obesity. *Journal of the American Medical Association*, **118**, 495–498.

Benedict, F. G. (1930) A helmet for use in clinical studies of gaseous metabolism. *New England Journal of Medicine*, **203**, 150–158.

Benn, R. T. (1971) Some mathematical properties of weight-for-height indices used as measures of adiposity. *British Journal of Preventive and Social Medicine*, **25**, 42–50.

Benoit, F. L., Martin, R. L. & Watten, R. H. (1965) Changes in body composition during weight reduction in obesity: balance studies comparing the effect of fasting and a ketogenic diet. *Annals of Internal Medicine*, **63**, 604–612.

Benzinger, T. H., Huebscher, R. G., Minard, D. & Kitzinger, C. (1958) Human calorimetry by means of the gradient principle. *Journal of Applied Physiology*, **12**, Supplement 1, 1–28.

Bernard, J. L. (1968) Rapid treatment of gross obesity by operant techniques. *Psychological Report*, **23**, 663–666.

Billewicz, W. Z. & Thomson, A. M. (1970) Body weight in parous women. *British Journal of Social and Preventive Medicine*, **24**, 97–104.

Binnie, C. C. (1977) Obesity in general practice. Ten year follow-up of obesity. *Journal of the Royal College of General Practitioners*, **27**, 492–495.

Bistrian, B. R. (1978) Clinical use of a protein-sparing modified fast. *Journal of the American Medical Association*, **240**, 2299–2302.

Bistrian, B. R., Blackburn, G. L. & Scrimshaw, N. S. (1975) Effect of mild infectious illness in nitrogen balance in patients on a modified fast. *American Journal of Clinical Nutrition*, **28**, 1044–1051.

Bistrian, B. R., Blackburn, G. L. & Stanbury, J. B. (1977b) Protein sparing modified fast in the management of Prader-Willi obesity. *New England Journal of Medicine*, **296**, 774–779.

Bistrian, B. R., Winterer, J., Blackburn, G. L., Young, V. & Sherman, M. (1977a) Effect of a protein-sparing diet and brief fast on nitrogen metabolism in mildly obese patients. *Journal of Laboratory and Clinical Medicine*, **89**, 1030–1035.

Bjorntorp, P. & Sjöström, L. (1979) Adipose tissue cellularity. *International Journal of Obesity*, **3**, 181–187.

Blackburn, G. L., Flatt, J. P., Clowes, G. H. A., O'Donnel, T. F. & Hensle, T. E. (1973) Protein sparing therapy during periods of starvation with sepsis or trauma. *Annals of Surgery*, **177**, 588–594.

Blackburn, M. W. & Calloway, D. H. (1976) Energy expenditure and consumption of mature, pregnant and lactating women. *Journal of the American Dietetic Association*, **69**, 29–37.

Blair, B. F. & Haines, L. W. (1966) Mortality experience according to build at higher durations. *Transactions of the Actuarial Society of America*, **18**, 35–41.

Blake, A. (1976) Group approach to weight control: behaviour modification, nutrition and health education. *Journal of the American Dietetic Association*, **69**, 645–649.

Blaxter, K. L., Brockway, J. M. & Boyne, A. W. (1972) A new method for estimating the heat production of animals. *Quarterly Journal of Experimental Physiology*, **57**, 60–72.

Blaza, S. E. (1980) Thermogenesis in lean and obese individuals. *PhD Thesis*, CNAA.

Blaza, S. E. & Garrow, J. S. (1980) The effect of anxiety on metabolic rate. *Proceedings of the Nutrition Society*, **39**, 13A.

Blundell, J. (1979) Hunger, appetite and satiety — constructs in search of identities. In *Nutrition and lifestyles*, ed. Turner, M. pp. 21–42. Applied Science Publishers, London.

Blundell, J. E. & Burridge, S. L. (1979) Control of feeding and the pychopharmacoogy of anorexic drugs. In: *The treatment of obesity*, ed. Munro, J. F. pp. 53–84. Lancaster, MTP Press.

Boddy, K., Hume, R., White, C., Pack, A., King, P. C., Weyers, E., Rowan, T. & Mills, E. (1976) The relation between potassium in body fluids and total body potassium in healthy and diabetic subjects. *Clinical Science and Molecular Medicine*, **50**, 455–461.

Bolden, K. J. (1975) Against the active treatment of obesity in general practice. *Update*, **2**, 339–348.

Bonjour, J. Ph., Welti, H. J. & Jéquier, E. (1976) Etude calorimetrique des consignes thermoregulatrices au declenchement de la sudation et au cours du cycle menstruel. *Journal de Physiologie* (Paris), **72**, 181–204.

Bolinger, R. E., Lukert, B. P., Brown, R. W., Guevara, L. & Steinberg, R. (1966) Metabolic balance of obese patients during fasting. *Archives of Internal Medicine* (Chicago), **118**, 3–8.

Booth, D. A. (1977) Satiety and appetite are conditioned reactions. *Psychosomatic Medicine*, **39**, 76–81.

Booth, D. A. (1978) First steps toward an integrated quantitative approach to human feeding and obesity with some implications for research into treatment. In *Recent advances in obesity research: 2*, ed. Bray, G. pp. 54–65. Newman, London.

Booth, D. A., Lee, M. & McAleavey, C. (1976) Acquired sensory control of satiation in man. *British Journal of Psychology*, **67**, 2, 137–147.

Borberg, C., Gillmer, M. D. G., Brunner, E. J., Gunn, P. J., Oakley, N. W. & Beard, R. W. (1980) Obesity in pregnancy: the effect of dietary advice. *Diabetes Care*, **3**, 476–481.

Borjeson, M. (1976) The aetiology of obesity in children. *Acta Paediatrica Scandinavica*, **65**, 279–287.

Bortz, W. M. (1969) A 500 pound weight loss. *American Journal of Medicine*, **47**, 325–331.

Bray, G. A. (ed.) (1979) Obesity in America. *National Institute of Health Publication* No. 79–358: US Department of Health Education & Welfare.

Bray, G. A., Barry, R. E., Benfield, J. R., Castelnuovo-Tedesco, P. & Rodin, J. (1976a) Intestinal bypass surgery for obesity decreases food intake and taste preferences. *American Journal of Clinical Nutrition*, **29**, 779–783.

Bray, G. A., Jordan, H. A. & Sims, E. A. H. (1976b) Evaluation of the obese patient. *Journal of the American Medical Association*, **235**, 1487–1491.

Bray, G. A., Raben, M. S., Londono, J. & Gallagher, T. F. (1971) Effects of triiodothyronine, growth hormone, and anabolic steroids on nitrogen excretion and oxygen consumption of obese patients. *Journal of Clinical Endocrinology*, **33**, 293–300.

Brewer, T. (1967) Human pregnancy nutrition: a clinical view. *Obstetrics and Gynecology*, **30**, 605–607.

Brook, C. G. D., Huntley, R. M. C. & Slack, J. (1975) Influence of heredity and environment in determination of skinfold thickness in children. *British Medical Journal*, **ii**, 719–721.

Brown, G. A., Bennetto, H. P., Miller, D. S., Rigby, M., Stock, M. J. & Stirling, J. L. (1977) A D.I.Y. human calorimeter for £100. *Proceedings of the Nutrition Society*, **36**, 13A.

Brownell, K. D. & Stunkard, A. J. (1978a) Behavior therapy and behavior change: uncertainties in programs for weight control. *Behavior Research and Therapy*, **16**, 301.

Brownell, K. D. & Stunkard, A. J. (1978b) Behavioural treatment of obesity in children. *American Journal of Diseases of Children*, **132**, 403–412.

Bruch, H. (1940) Obesity in childhood: III. Physiologic and psychologic aspects of the food intake of obese children. *American Journal of Diseases of Children*, **59**, 739–781.

Bruch, H. (1961) Conceptual confusion in eating disorders. *Journal of Nervous and Mental Disorders*, **133**, 46–54.

Bruch, H. (1974) *Eating disorders: obesity, anorexia nervosa, and the person within*, p. 396. London, Routledge & Kegan Paul.

Bryson, E., Doré, C. & Garrow, J. S. (1979) Wholemeal bread and satiety. *Lancet*, **ii**, 260–261.

Buchwald, H. (1980) True informed consent in surgical treatment of morbid obesity: the current case for both jejunoileal and gastric bypass. *American Journal of Clinical Nutrition*, **33**, 482–494.

Buckwalter, J. A. (1980) Morbid obesity: good and poor results of jejunoileal and gastric bypass. *American Journal of Clinical Nutrition*, **33**, 476–480.

Burch, P. R. J. & Spiers, F. W. (1953) Measurements of the γ radiation from the human body. *Nature* (London), **172**, 519–521.

Burke, B. S. (1947) The dietary history as a tool in research. *Journal of the American Dietetic Association*, **23**, 1041–1046.

Burman, K. D., Dimond, R. C., Harvey, G. S., O'Brian, J. T., Georges, L. P., Bruton, J., Wright, F. D. & Wartofsky, L. (1979) Glucose modulation of alterations in serum iodothyronine concentrations induced by fasting. *Metabolism*, **28**, 291–299.

Buss, D. H. & Ruck, N. F. (1977) The aminoacid pattern of the British Diet. *Journal of Human Nutrition*, **31**, 165–169.

Cabanac, M. & Duclaux, R. (1970) Obesity: absence of satiety aversion to sucrose. *Science*, **168**, 496–497.

Cabanac, M. & Rabe, E. F. (1976) Influence of a monotonous food on body weight regulation in humans. *Physiology and Behaviour*, **17**, 675–678.

Cahill, G. F. (1978) Obesity and diabetes. In *Recent advances in obesity research: 2*, ed. Bray, G. pp. 101–110. Newman Publishing, London.

Calloway, D. H. & Spector, H. (1954) Nitrogen balance as related to caloric and protein intake in active young men. *American Journal of Clinical Nutrition*, **2**, 405–411.

Campbell, R. G., Hashim, S. A. & van Itallie, T. B. (1971) Nutritive density and food intake in man. *New England Journal of Medicine*, **285**, 1402–1407.

Carey, M. E., Pilkington, T. R. E. & Titterington, E. (1962) Ketosis and body weight. *Lancet*, **ii**, 1189–1190.

Charney, E., Goodman, H. C., McBride, M., Lyon, B. & Pratt, R. (1976) Childhood antecedents of adult obesity. *New England Journal of Medicine*, **295**, 6–9.

Chave, S. P., Morris, J. N., Moss, S. & Semmence, A. M. (1978) Vigorous exercise in leisure time and death rate: a study of male civil servants. *Journal of Epidemiology and Community Health*, **32**, 239–243.

Choksi, R., Bower, P. B., Pollard, V. & Mankad, V. N. (1980) Evaluation of a programme for weight control for obese children and adolescents. *Illinois Medical Journal*, **157**, 232–235.

Coates, T. J. & Thorensen, C. E. (1978) Treating obesity in children and adolescents: A review. *American Journal of Public Health*, **68**, 143–152.

Cochrane, A. L., Moore, F., Baker, I. A. & Haley, T. J. L. (1980) Mortality in two random samples of women aged 55–64 followed up for 20 years. *British Medical Journal*, **280**, 1131–1133.

Coll, M., Meyer, A. & Stunkard, A. J. (1979) Obesity and food choices in public places. *Archives of General Psychiatry*, **36**, 795–797.

Combes, R., Altomare, E., Tramoni, M. & Vague, J. (1979) Obesity and menstrual disorder. In: *Medical complications of obesity*, ed. Mancini, M., Lewis, B. & Contaldo, F. pp. 285–288. London, Academic Press.

Cook, L. (1978) Relationship of blood pressure, serum cholesterol, smoking habit, relative weight and ECG abnormalities to incidence of major coronary events: final report of the pooling project. Edited for the pooling project research group by L. P. Cook. *Journal of Chronic Diseases*, **31**, 201–306.

Coupar, A. M. & Kennedy, T. (1980) Running a weight control group: experiences of a psychologist and a general practitioner. *Journal of the Royal College of General Practitioners*, **30**, 41–48.

Craddock, D. (1973) *Obesity and its management*, p. 205. Edinburgh, Churchill Livingstone.

Crisp, A. H. (1973) The nature of primary anorexia nervosa. In *Anorexia nervosa and obesity*, ed. Robertson, R. F. pp. 18–30. Edinburgh, Royal College of Physicians.

Crisp, A. H. & McGuiness, B. (1976) Jolly fat: relation between obesity and psychoneurosis in general population. *British Medical Journal*, **i**, 7–9.

Cummings, J. H., Southgate, D. A. T., Branch, W. J., Wiggins, H. S., Houston, H., Jenkins, D. J. A., Jivraj, T. & Hill, M. J. (1979) The digestion of pectin in the human gut and its effect on calcium absorption and large bowel function. *British Journal of Nutrition*, **41**, 477–485.

Dahlkoetter, J., Callaghan, E. J. & Linton, J. (1979) Obesity and the unbalanced energy equation: exercise versus eating habit change. *Journal of Consulting and Clinical Psychology*, **47**, 898–905.

Dahms, W. T., Molitch, M. E., Bray, G. A., Greenway, F. L., Atkinson, R. L. & Hamilton, K. (1978) Treatment of obesity: cost-benefit assessment of behavioural therapy, placebo, and two anorectic drugs. *American Journal of Clinical Nutrition*, **31**, 774–778.

Dauncey, J. M. (1980) Metabolic effects of altering the 24 h energy intake in man, using direct and indirect calorimetry. *British Journal of Nutrition*, **43**, 257–270.

Dauncey, M. J., Murgatroyd, P. R. & Cole, T. J. (1978) A human calorimeter for the direct and indirect measurement of 24 hour energy expenditure. *British Journal of Nutrition*, **39**, 557–566.

Davidson, S., Passmore, R., Brock, J. F. & Truswell, A. S. (1979) *Human Nutrition and Dietetics*, 7th edition, Churchill Livingstone, Edinburgh.

DeHaven, J., Sherwin, R., Hendler, R. & Felig, P. (1980) Nitrogen and sodium balance and sympathetic-nervous-system activity in obese subjects treated with a low-calorie protein or mixed diet. *New England Journal of Medicine*, **302**, 477–482.

DeJong, W. (1980) The stigma of obesity: the consequences of naive assumptions concerning the causes of physical deviance. *Journal of Health and Social Behaviour*, **20**, 75–87.

Department of Health and Social Security (1969) *Recommended intakes of nutrients for the United Kingdom*. HMSO, London.

Department of Health and Social Security (1979) *Recommended daily amounts of food energy and nutrients for groups of people in the United Kingdom*, p. 27. HMSO, London.

Dickerson, J. W. T. & Widdowson, E. M. (1960) Chemical changes in skeletal muscle during development. *Biochemical Journal*, **74**, 247–257.

Dine, M. S., Gartside, P. S., Glueck, C. J., Rheines, L., Greene, G. & Khoury, P. (1979) Where do the heaviest children come from? A prospective study of white children from birth to 5 years of age. *Pediatrics*, **63**, 1–7.

Dixon, A. S. & Henderson, D. (1973) Prescribing for osteoarthrosis. *Prescribers Journal*, **13**, 41–49.

Donald, D. W. A. (1973) Mortality rates among the overweight. In *Anorexia and Obesity*, ed. Robertson, R. F. pp. 63–70. Royal College of Physicians, Edinburgh.

Doré, C., Hesp, R., Wilkins, D. & Garrow, J. S. (1981) A standard for resting metabolic rate in obese women. (in preparation)

Douglas, J. G., Ford, M. J. & Munro, J. F. (1979) Obesity — to treat or not to treat. *Scottish Medical Journal*, **24**, 72–75.

Drenick, E. J. (1976) Weight reduction by prolonged fasting. In *Obesity in perspective*, ed. Bray, G. pp. 341–360. Fogarty International Center, U.S. Government Printing House, Washington, D.C.

Drenick, E. J. & Hargis, H,. W. (1978) Jaw wiring for weight reduction. *Obesity and Bariatric Medicine*, **7**, 210–213.

Dublin, L. I. (1953) Relation of obesity to longevity. *New England Journal of Medicine*, **248**, 971–974.

Dubois, D. D. & Fizer, M. E. (1978) Psychosexual dysfunction in patients with immobilized jaws. *Oral Surgery*, **46**, 506–510.

Dubois, S., Hill, D. E. & Beaton, G. H. (1979) An examination of factors believed to be associated with infantile obesity. *American Journal of Clinical Nutrition*, **32**, 1997–2004.

Durnin, J. V. G. A. & McKillop, F. M. (1978) The relationship between body build in infancy and percentage body fat in adolescence: a 14 year follow-up of 102 infants. *Proceedings of the Nutrition Society*, **37**, 81A.

Durnin, J. V. G. A. & Womersley, J. (1974) Body fat assessed from body density and its estimation from skinfold thickness: measurement on 481 men and women from 16–72 years. *British Journal of Nutrition*, **32**, 77–97.

Durrant, M. L. (1980) The effect of changes in preload energy content on energy intake of obese and lean subjects. *Proceedings of the Nutrition Society*, **39**, 87A.

Durrant, M. & Ashwell, M. (1979) Hunger and appetite characteristics of obese patients on an inpatient weight reduction programme. *International Journal of Obesity*, **3**, 91–92.

Durrant, M. L., Garrow, J. S., Royston, P., Stalley, S. F., Sunkin, S. and Warwick, P. (1980) Factors influencing the composition of the weight lost by obese patients on a reducing diet. *British Journal of Nutrition*, **44**, 275–285.

Durrant, M. & Mann, S. (1977) Investigations into patient responses to feeding low- and high-energy foods. *Proceedings of the Nutrition Society*, **36**, 113A.

Durrant, M. & Wloch, R. (1979) The effect of palatability on energy intake in two obese women. *Proceedings of the Nutrition Society*, **38**, 37A.

Dwyer, J. T. & Berman, E. M. (1978) Battling the bulge: a continuing struggle. Two-year follow-up of successful losers in a commercial dieting concern. In *Recent Advances in Obesity Research: 2*, ed. Bray, G. pp. 277–294. London, Newman Publishing.

Dyer, A. R., Stamler, J., Berkson, D. M. & Lindberg, H. A. (1975) Relationship of relative weight and body mass index to 14 year mortality in the Chicago Peoples Gas Company study. *Journal of Chronic Diseases*, **28**, 109–123.

Edholm, O. G. (1977) Energy balance in man. *Journal of Human Nutrition*, **31**, 413–432.

Edholm, O. G., Adam, J. M., Healy, M. J. R., Wolff, H. S., Goldsmith, R. & Best, T. W. (1970) Food intake and energy expenditure of army recruits. *British Journal of Nutrition*, **24**, 1091–1107.

Edholm, O. G., Fletcher, J. G., Widdowson, E. M. & McCance, R. A. (1955) The energy expenditure and food intake of individual men. *British Journal of Nutrition*, **9**, 286–300.

Edwards, H. T., Thorndike, A. & Dill, D. B. (1935) The energy requirement in strenuous muscular exercise. *New England Journal of Medicine*, **213**, 532–535.

Edwards, L. E., Dickes, W. F., Alton, I. R. & Hakanson, E. Y. (1978) Pregnancy in the massively obese: course outcome and obesity prognosis for the infant. *American Journal of Obstetrics and Gynecology*, **131**, 479–483.

Efiong, E. I. (1975) Pregnancy in the overweight Nigerian. *British Journal of Obstetrics and Gynaecology*, **82**, 903–906.

Eid, E. E. (1970) Follow-up study of physical growth of children who had excessive weight gain in first six months of life. *British Medical Journal*, **ii**, 74–76.

Evans, E. & Miller, D. S. (1977) The effect of ephidrene on the oxygen consumption of fed and fasted subjects. *Proceedings of the Nutrition Society*, **36**, 136A.

Fabry, P. (1973) Food intake pattern and energy balance. In *Energy balance in man*, ed. Apfelbaum, M. pp. 297–303. Paris, Masson.

Faloon, W. W., Flood, M. S., Aroesty, S. & Sherman, C. D. (1980) Assessment of jejunoileostomy for obesity — some observations since 1976. *American Journal of Clinical Nutrition*, **33**, 431–439.

FAO/WHO (1973) *Energy and protein requirements*. WHO Technical Report Series No. 522, FAO, Rome.

Farquhar, J. W. (1978) The Stanford Three-Community Study: Health education for cardiovascular risk prevention. In: *Recent Advances in Obesity Research: 2*, ed. Bray, G. pp. 313–320. London, Newman Publishing.

Fentem, P. H. (1978) Advice on exercise. *British Medical Journal*, **ii**, 429.

Fisch, R. O., Bilek, M. K. & Ulstrom, R. (1975) Obesity and leanness at birth and their relationship to body habitus in later childhood. *Pediatrics*, **56**, 521–528.

Flatt, J. P. & Blackburn, G. L. (1974) Metabolic fuel regulatory system: implications for protein-sparing therapies during caloric deprivation and disease. American Journal of Clinical Nutrition, **27**, 175–187.

Forbes, G. B. & Drenick, E. J. (1979) Loss of body nitrogen on fasting. *American Journal of Clinical Nutrition*, **32**, 1570–1574.

Forbes, G. B. & Lewis, A. M. (1956) Total sodium, potassium and chloride in adult man. *Journal of Clinical Investigation*, **35**, 596–600.

Forbes, R. M., Cooper, A. R. & Mitchell, H. H. (1953) The composition of the adult human body as determined by chemical analysis. *Journal of Biological Chemistry*, **203**, 359–366.

Forbes, R. M., Mitchell, H. H. & Cooper, A. R. (1956) Further studies on the gross composition and mineral elements of the adult human body. *Journal of Biological Chemistry*, **223**, 969–875.

Fordyce, G. L., Garrow, J. S., Kark, A. E. & Stalley, S. F. (1979) Jaw wiring and gastric bypass in the treatment of severe obesity. *Obesity and Bariatric Medicine*, **8**, 14–17.

Foreyt, J. P. & Kennedy, W. A. (1971) Treatment of overweight by aversion therapy. *Behaviour Research and Therapy*, **9**, 29–34.

Foss, M. L., Lampman, R. M. & Schteingart, D. (1976) Physical training program for rehabilitating extremely obese patients. *Archives of Physical Medicine and Rehabilitation*, **57**, 425–429.

Fox, F. W. (1973) The enigma of obesity. *Lancet*, **ii**, 1487–1488.

Fuller, J. H., Shipley, M. J., Rose, G., Jarrett, R. J. & Keen, H. (1980) Coronary-heart- disease risk and impaired glucose tolerance. *Lancet*, **i**, 1373–1376.

Garattini, S. and Samanin, R. (1976) Anorectic drugs and brain neurotransmitters. In: *Appetite and food intake*, ed. Silverstone, T. pp. 83–108. Berlin, Dahlem Konferenzen.

Garby, L. & Lammert, O. (1977) Effect of the preceding day's energy intake on the total energy cost of light exercise. *Acta Physiologica Scandinavica*, **101**, 411–417.

Garn, S. M. & Clark, D. C. (1976) Trends in fatness and the origins of obesity. *Pediatrics*, **57**, 443–456.

Garn, S. M. & Cole, P. E. (1980) Do the obese remain obese and the lean remain lean? *American Journal of Public health*, **70**, 351–353.

Garrow, J. S. (1974) *Energy balance and obesity in man*, pp. 362, North Holland Publishing Co., Amsterdam.

Garrow, J. S. (1975) A survey of three slimming and weight control organisations in the U.K. In *Recent advances in obesity Research: 1*, ed. Howard, A., pp. 301–304. London. Newman Publishing.

Garrow, J. S. (1978a) *Energy balance and obesity in man*, p. 243. 2nd edn. Elsevier, Amsterdam.

Garrow, J. S. (1978b) The regulation of energy expenditure in man. In *Recent advances in obesity research: 2*, ed. Bray, G., pp. 200–210. London: Newman Publishing.

Garrow, J. S. (1979a) Weight penalties. *British Medical Journal*, **ii**, 1171–1172.

Garrow, J. S. (1979b) Lower energy expenditure as an aggravating factor in crippling obesity. In *Medical complications of obesity*, ed. Mancini, M., Lewis, B. & Contaldo, F.pp. 295–300. Academic Press, London.

Garrow, J. S. (1980) Combined medical-surgical approaches to treatment of obesity. *American Journal of Clinical Nutrition*, **33**, 425–430.

Garrow, J. S. & Gardiner, G. T. (1981) Maintenance of weight loss in obese patients after jaw wiring. *British Medical Journal*, **282**, 858–860.

Garrow, J. S. & Hawes, S. F. (1972) The role of aminoacid oxidation in causing 'specific dynamic action' in man. *British Journal of Nutrition*, **27**, 2211–219.

Garrow, J. S. & Stalley, S. F. (1975) Is there a set point for human body weight? *Proceedings of the Nutrition Society*, **34**, 84A.

Garrow, J. S. & Stalley, S. F. (1977) Cognitive thresholds and human body weight. *Proceedings of the Nutrition Society*, **36**, 18A.

Garrow, J. S. & Wright, D. (1980) Burning off unwanted energy. *Lancet*, **i**, 377.

Garrow, J. S., Belton, E. A. & Daniels, A. (1972) A controlled investigation of the 'glycolyptic' action of fenfluramine. *Lancet*, **ii**, 559–561.

Garrow, J. S., Blaza, S. E., Warwick, P. M. & Ashwell, M. A. (1980) Predisposition to obesity. *Lancet,* **i,** 1103–1104.

Garrow, J. S., Murgatroyd, P., Toft, R. & Warwick, P. (1977) A direct calorimeter for clinical use. *Journal of Physiology* (London), **267,** 16p.

Garrow, J. S., Durrant, M. L., Mann, S., Stalley, S. F. & Warwick, P. (1978) Factors determining weight loss in obese patients in a metabolic ward. *International Journal of Obesity,* **2,** 441–447.

Garrow, J. S., Durrant, M. L., Blaza, S., Wilkins, D., Royston, P. & Sunkin, S. 1981) The effect of meal frequency and protein concentration on the composition of the weight lost by obese women. *British Journal of Nutrition.*

Garrow, J. S., Stalley, S., Diethelm, R., Pittet, Ph., Hesp, R. & Halliday, D. (1979) A new method for measuring the body density of obese adults. *British Journal of Nutrition,* **42,** 173–183.

Garry, R. C., Passmore, R., Warnock, G. M. & Durnin, J. V. G. A. (1955) *Studies on expenditure of energy and consumption of food by miners and clerks, Fife, Scotland, 1952.* Medical Research Council, Special Report Series No. 289, H.M.S.O London. pp. 70.

Genuth, S. M. (1973) Plasma insulin and glucose profiles in normal, obese, and diabetic persons. *Annals of Internal Medicine,* **79,** 812–822.

Genuth, S. (1979) Supplemented fasting in the treatment of obesity and diabetes. *American Journal of Clinical Nutrition,* **32,** 2579–2586.

Gilder, H., Cornell, G. N., Grafe, W. R., Macfarlane, J. R., Asaph, J. W., Stubenbord, W. T., Watkins, G. M., Rees, J. R. & Thorbjarnarson, B. (1967) Components of weight loss in obese patients subjected to prolonged starvation. *Journal of Applied Physiology,* **23,** 304–310.

Girandola, R. N. (1976) Body composition changes in women: effects of high and low exercise intensities. *Archives of Physical Medicine and Rehabilitation,* **57,** 297–299.

Gold, R. M. (1973) Hypothalamic obesity: the myth of the ventromedial nucleus. *Science,* **182,** 488–490.

Gomez, C. A. (1980) Gastroplasty in the surgical treatment of morbid obesity. *American Journal of Clinical Nutrition,* **33,** 406–415.

Goodner, C. J. & Ogilvie, J. T. (1974) Homeostasis of body weight in a diabetes clinic population. *Diabetes,* **23,** 318–326.

Gordon, T. & Kannel, W. B. (1973) The effects of overweight on cardiovascular disease. *Geriatrics,* **28,** 80–88.

Goss, A. N. (1979) Management of patients with jaws wired for obesity. *British Dental Journal,* **146,** 335–339.

Götestam, K. G. (1979) A three-year follow-up of a behavioural treatment for obesity. *Addictive Behaviour,* **4,** 179–183.

Gray, H. & Kallenbach, D. C. (1939) Obesity treatment: results in 212 outpatients. *Journal of the American Dietetic Association,* **15,** 239–245.

Grimes, D. S. & Goddard, J. (1977) Gastric emptying of wholemeal and white bread *Gut,* **18,** 725–729.

Grinker, J. (1978) Obesity and sweet taste. *American Journal of Clinical Nutrition,* **31,** 1078–1087.

Groen, J. J., Tijong, K. B., Koster, M., Willebrands, A. F. Verdonck, G. & Pierloot, M. (1962) The influence of nutrition and ways of life on blood cholesterol and the prevalence of hypertension and coronorary heart disease among Trappist and Benedictine monks. *American Journal of Clinical Nutrition,* **10,** 456–470.

Gurr, M. I. & Kirtland, J. (1978a) Adipose tissue cellularity: a review. 1. Techniques for studying cellularity. *International Journal of Obesity,* **2,** 401–427.

Gurr, M. I. & Kirtland, J. (1978b) Adipost tissue cellularity: a review. 2. The relationship between cellularity and obesity. *International Journal of Obesity,* **3,** 15–55.

Gurr, M. I., Robinson, M. P. & Maltby, D. (1979) A simple and cheap respiration chamber for long-term studies of energy expenditure in human beings. *Proceedings of the Nutrition Society*, **38**, 64A.

Gwinup, G. (1975) Effect of exercise alone on the weight of obese women. *Archives of Internal Medicine*, **135**, 676–680.

Hall, S. M., Hall, R. G., DeBoer, G. & O'Kulitch, P. (1977) Self and external management compared with psychotherapy in the control of obesity. *Behaviour Research and Therapy*, **15**, 89–95.

Hallberg, D. (1980) A survey of surgical techniques for treatment of obesity and a remark on the bilio-intestinal bypass method. *American Journal of Clinical Nutrition*, **33**, 499–501.

Halliday, D., Hesp, R., Stalley, S. F., Warwick, P., Altman, D. G. & Garrow, J. S. (1979) Resting metabolic rate, weight, surface area and body composition in obese women. *International Journal of Obesity*, **3**, 1–6.

Halliday, D. & Miller, A. G. (1977) Precise measurement of total body water using trace quantities of deuterium oxide. *Biomedical Mass Spectrometry*, **4**, 82–87.

Hammar, S. L., Campbell, M. M., Campbell, V. A., Moores, N. L., Sareen, C., Garcis, F. J. & Lucas, B. (1972) An interdisciplinary study of adolescent obesity. *Journal of Pediatrics*, **80**, 373–383.

Harding, P. E. (1980) Jaw wiring for obesity. *Lancet*, **i**, 534–535.

Hartz, A. J., Barboriak, P. N., Wong, A., Katayama, K. P. & Rimm, A. A. (1979) The association of obesity with infertility and menstrual abnormalities in women. *International Journal of Obesity*, **3**, 57–73.

Hartz, A. J. & Rimm, A. A. (1980) Natural history of obesity in 6,946 women between 50 and 59 years of age. *American Journal of Public Health*, **70**, 385–388.

Hashim, S. A. & van Itallie, T. B. (1965) Studies in normal and obese subjects with a monitored food dispensing service. *Annals of the New York Academy of Sciences*, **131**, 654–661.

Hawk, L. J. & Brook, C. G. D. (1979) Influence of body fatness in childhood on fatness in adult life. *British Medical Journal*, **i**, 151–152.

Heaton, K. W. (1973) Food fibre as an obstacle to energy intake. *Lancet*, **ii**, 1418–1421.

Hervey, G. R. (1969) Regulation of energy balance. *Nature* (London), **222**, 629–631.

Hill, G. L., Bradley, J. A., Collins, J. P., McCarthy, I., Oxby, C. B. & Burkinshaw, L. (1978) Fat-free body mass from skinfold thickness: a close relationship with total body nitrogen. *British Journal of Nutrition*, **39**, 403–405.

Hirsch, J. (1975) Cell number and size as a determinant of subsequent obesity. In *Childhood Obesity*, ed. Winick, M., pp. 15–21. New York: John Wiley.

Hirsch, J. & Batchelor, B. (1976) Adipose tissue cellularity in human obesity. *Clinics in Endocrinology and Metabolism*, **5**, 299–311.

Hirsch, J. & Gallian, E. (1968) Methods for the determination of adipose cell size in man and animals. *Journal of Lipid Research*, **9**, 110–119.

Hood, C. E. A., Goodhart, J. M., Fletcher, R. F., Gloster, J., Bertrand, P. V. & Crooke, A. C. (1970) Observations on obese patients eating isocaloric reducing diets with varying proportions of carbohydrate. *British Journal of Nutrition*, **24**, 39–44.

Howard, A. N. & Baird, I. McL. (1977) A long-term evaluation of very low calorie semisynthetic diets: an inpatient/outpatient study with egg albumin as the protein source. *International Journal of Obesity*, **1**, 63–78.

Howard, A. N., Grant, A., Edwards, O., Littlewood, E. R. & Baird, I. McL. (1978) The treatment of obesity with a very-low-calorie liquid-formula diet: an inpatient/ outpatient comparison using skimmed-milk protein as the chief protein source. *International Journal of Obesity*, **2**, 321–332.

Humphrey, S. J. E. & Wolff, H. S. (1977) The oxylog. *Journal of Physiology* (London), **267**, 12p.

Hunt, J. N., Cash, R. & Newland, P. (1975) Energy density of food, gastric emptying, and obesity. *Lancet*, **ii**, 905–906.

Hunt, J. N., Cash, R. & Newland, P. (1978) Energy density of food, gastric emptying, and obesity. *American Journal of Clinical Nutrition*, 31 (10 Suppl) S259–S260.

Hytten, F. E. (1979) Restriction of weight gain in pregnancy: is it justified? *Journal of Human Nutrition*, 33, 461–463.

Hytten, F. E. (1980) Nutrition, in *Clinical physiology in obstetrics*, Hytten, F. & G. Chamberlain, G. pp. 163–192. Oxford, Blackwell Scientific.

Hytten, F. E. & Leitch, I. (1964) *The physiology of human pregnancy*. p. 463. Oxford, Blackwell.

James, W. P. T. (1976) Compiler. *Research on Obesity: a report of the DHSS/MRC Group*. p. 94. Her Majesty's Stationery Office. London.

James, W. P. T. (1981) Depressed thermogenesis in animal and human obesity. In *Recent Advances in Obesity Research: 3*, eds. Howard, A. N., Björntorp, O. & Cairella, M. London: John Libbey.

Jeejeebhoy, K. N. (1976) Total parenteral nutrition. *Annals of the Royal College of Physicians, Canada*, 9, 287–300.

Jeffery, R. W., Thompson, P. D. & Wing, R. R. (1978) Effects on weight reduction of strong monetary contracts for calorie restriction or weight loss. *Behaviour Research and Therapy*, 16, 363–369.

Johnson, P. R., Stern, J. S., Greenwood, M. R. C., Zucker, L. M. & Hirsch, J. (1973) Effect of early nutrition on adipose cellularity and pancreatic insulin release in the Zucker rat. *Journal of Nutrition*, 103, 738–743.

Johnson, R. E. (1980) Techniques for measuring gas exchange. In *Assessment of energy metabolism in health and disease*, ed. Kinney, J. pp. 32–35. First Ross Conference on Medical Research, Columbus, Ohio.

Jolliffe, N. & Alpert, E. (1951) The 'performance index' as a method for estimating effectiveness of reducing regimens. *Postgraduate Medicine*, 9, 106–115.

Jourdan, M., Margen, S. & Bradfield, R. B. (1974) Protein-sparing effects in obese women fed low calorie diets. *American Journal of Clinical Nutrition*, 27, 3–12.

Jung, R. T., Gurr, M. I., Robinson, M. P. & James, W. P. T. (1978) Does adipocyte hypercellularity in obesity exist? *British Medical Journal*, ii, 319–321.

Kalucy, R. S. (1980) Drug-induced weight gain. *Drugs*, 19, 268–278.

Kannel, W. B. & Sorlie, P. (1979) Some health benefits of physical activity. *Archives of Internal Medicine*, 139, 857–861.

Kempner, W., Newborg, B. C., Peschel, R. L. & Skyler, J. S. (1975) Treatment of massive obesity with rice/reduction diet programme. *Archives of Internal Medicine*, 135, 1575–1584.

Kennedy, I. (1980) Consumerism in the doctor-patient relationship. *The Listener*, 104, 777–780.

Kennedy, G. C. (1950) The hypothalamic control of food intake in rats. *Proceedings of the Royal Society, London, (B)*, 137, 535–549.

Keys, A. (1970) Coronary heart disease in seven countries. *Circulation*, 41, Suppl. 1.

Keys, A., Aravanis, C., Blackburn, H., van Buchem, F. S. P., Buzina, R., Djordjevic, B. S., Fidanza, F., Karvonen, M. J., Menotti, A., Puddu, V. & Taylor, H. L. (1972) Coronary heart disease: overweight and obesity as risk factors. *Annals of Internal Medicine*, 77, 15–27.

Keys, A., Brozek, J., Henschel, A., Mickelson, O. & Taylor, H. L. (1950) *The Biology of Human Starvation*, p. 831. University of Minnesota Press, Minneapolis.

Kinney, J. M. (1980) The application of indirect calorimetry to clinical studies. In *Assessment of energy metabolism in health and disease*, ed. Kinney, J. pp. 42–48. First Ross Conference on Medical Research, Columbus, Ohio.

Knittle, J. L., Ginsberg-Fellner, F. & Brown, R. E. (1977) Adipose tissue development in man. *American Journal of Clinical Nutrition*, 30, 762–766.

Konishi, F. & Harrison, S. L. (1977) Body weight gain equivalents of selected foods. *Journal of the American Dietetic Association*, 70, 365–368.

Kopp, W. K. (1975) Problems with jaw fixation for weight control. *Journal of Oral Surgery*, **33**, 6.

Kral, J. G. (1980) Effects of truncal vagotomy on body weight and hyperinsulinaemia in morbid obesity. *Americancan Journal of Clinical Nutrition*, **33**, 416–419.

Krotkiewski, M., Sjöström, L., Björntorp, P., Carlgren, G., Garellick, G. & Smith, U. (1977) Adipose tissue cellularity in relation to prognosis for weight reduction. *International Journal of Obesity*, **1**, 395–416.

LaPorte, R. E., Kuller, L. H., Kupfer, D. J., McPartland, R. J., Matthews, G. & Caspersen, C. (1979) An objective measure of physical activity for epidemiological research. *American Journal of Epidemiology*, **109**, 158–168.

Leeds, A. R. (1979) Dietary management of diabetes in adults. *Proceedings of the Nutrition Society*, **38**, 365–371.

Lesser, G. T., Deutsch, S. & Markofsky, J. (1971) Use of independent measurement of body fat to evaluate overweight and underweight. *Metabolism*, **20**, 792–804.

Levitz, L. S. & Jordan, H. A. (1973) Manual for the analysis of energy intake and expenditure. In *Obesity in perspective*, ed. Bray, G. A., Vol. 2, Part 1, Appendix V. U.S. Government Printing Office, Washington, D.C.

Lew, E. A. & Garfinkel, L. (1979) Variations in mortality by weight among 750 000 men and women. *Journal of Chronic Diseases*, **32**, 563–576.

Lewis, S., Haskell, W. L., Wood, P. D., Manoogian, N., Bailey, J. E. & Pereira, M. B. (1976) Effects of physical activity on weight reduction in obese middle-aged women. *American Journal of Clinical Nutrition*, **29**, 151–156.

Lindstrom, L. L., Balch, P. & Reese, S. (1976) In person versus telephone treatment for obesity. *Journal of Behaviour Therapy & Experimental Psychiatry*, **7**, 367–369.

Lloyd, J. K., Wolff, O. H. & Whelen, W. S. (1961) Childhood obesity: a long-term study of height and weight. *British Medical Journal*, **ii**, 145–148.

Loro, A. D. Jr., Fisher, E. B. Jr. & Levenkron, J. C. (1979) Comparison of established and innovative weight-reduction procedures. *Journal of Applied Behaviour Analysis*, **12**, 141–145.

Maagøe, H. & Morgensen, E. F. (1970) Effect of treatment on obesity: a follow-up of material treated with complete starvation. *Danish Medical Bulletin*, **17**, 206–209.

Macnair, A. L. (1979) Burning off unwanted energy. *Lancet*, **ii**, 1300.

Maeder, E. C., Barno, A., Mecklenberg, F. (1975) Obesity: a maternal high risk factor. *Obstetrics and Gynecology*, **45**, 669–671.

Mahoney, M. J. (1974) Self-reward and self-monitoring techniques for weight control. *Behaviour Therapy*, **5**, 48–57.

Mann, G. V. (1977) Diet and obesity. *New England Journal of Medicine*, **296**, 812.

Mann, G. V. (1974) The influence of obesity on health. *New England Journal of Medicine*, **291**, 178–185, & 226–232.

Marliss, E. B. (1978) The physiology of fasting and semi-starvation: roles of 'caloristat' and 'aminostat' mechanisms. In *Recent Advances in Obesity Research 2* ed. Bray, G., pp. 345–358. Newman Publishing, London.

Marliss, E. B., Murray, F. T. & Nakhooda, A. F. (1978) The metabolic response to hypocaloric protein diet in obese man. *Journal of Clinical Investigation*, **62**, 468–479.

Marr, J. W. (1971) Individual dietary surveys: Purposes and Methods. *World Review Nutrition Dietetics*, **13**, 105–164.

Mason, E. (1970) Obesity in pet dogs. *Vetinary Record*, **86**, 612–616.

Mason, E. E. & Ito, C. (1969) Gastric Bypass. *Annals of Surgery*, **170**, 329–336.

Mason, E. E., Printen, K. J., Blommers, T. J., Lewis, J. W. & Scott, D. H. (1980) Gastric bypass in morbid obesity. *American Journal of Clinical Nutrition*, **33**, 395–405

Mayer, J., Marshall, N. B., Vitale, J. J., Christensen, J. H., Mashayekhi, M. B. & Stare, F. J. (1954) Exercise, food intake and body weight in normal rats and genetically obese adult mice. *American Journal of physiology*, 177, 544–548.

Mayer, J., Roy, P. & Mitra, K. P. (1956) Relation between caloric intake, body weight and physical work: studies in an industrial male population in West Bengal. *American Journal of Clinical Nutrition*, 4, 169–175.

McKeown, T. (1970) Prenatal and early postnatal influences on measured intelligence. *British Medical Journal*, iii, 63–67.

McMichael, J. (1979) Fats and atheroma: an inquest. *British Medical Journal*, i, 173–175.

Meade, C. J., Ashwell, M. & Sowter, C. (1979) Is genetically transmitted obesity due to an adipose tissue defect? *Proceedings of the Royal Society, London, B*, 205, 395–410.

Mellbin, T. & Vuille, J. C. (1973) Physical development at 7 years of age in relation to velocity of weight gain in infancy with special reference to incidence of overweight. *British Journal of Preventive and Social Medicine*, 27, 225–235.

Meyer, V. & Crisp, A. H. (1964) Aversion therapy in two cases of obesity. *Behaviour Research and Therapy*, 2, 134–147.

Miall, W. S. & Chinn, S. (1973) Blood pressure and ageing; results of a 15–17 year follow-up study in South Wales. *Clinical Science and Molecular Medicine*, 45, 23S–33S.

Miller, D. S., Mumford, P. & Stock, M. J. (1967) Gluttony 2. Thermogenesis in overeating Man. *American Journal of Clinical Nutrition*, 20, 1223–1229.

Miller, D. S. & Wise, A. (1975) Exercise and dietary-induced thermogenesis. *Lancet*, i, 1290.

Miller, M. M. (1974) Hypnoaversion in the treatment of obesity. *Journal of the National Medical Association*, 66, 480–481.

Miller, N. E., Rao, S., Lewis, B., Bjørsvik, G., Myhre, K. & Mjøs, O. D. (1979) High-density lipoprotein and physical activity. *Lancet*, i, 111.

Milvy, P., Forbes, W. F. & Brown, K. S. (1977) A critical review of epidemiological studies of physical activity. *Annals of the New York Academy of Sciences*, 301, 519–549.

Ministry of Agriculture, Fisheries and Food (1978) *Household Food Consumption and Expenditure: 1977*. HMSO, London.

Mitchell, H. H., Hamilton, T. S., Steggerda, F. R. & Bean, H. W. (1945) The chemical composition of the adult human body and its bearing on the biochemistry of growth. *Journal of Biological Chemistry*, 158, 625–637.

Moffitt, P. (1980) Physical training and coronary risk factors. *British Medical Journal*, 281, 453.

Moore, R., Grant, A. M., Howard, A. N. & Mills, I. H. (1980) Treatment of obesity with triiodothyronine and a very-low-calorie liquid formula diet. *Lancet*, i, 223–226.

Morris, J. N. (1980) Physical training and coronary risk factors. *British Medical Journal*, 281, 564.

Morris, J. N., Everitt, M. G., Pollard, R., Chave, S. P. W. & Semmence, A. M. (1980) Vigorous exercise in leisure-time: protection against coronary heart disease. *Lancet*, ii, 1207–1210.

Morris, J. N., Marr, J. W. & Clayton, D. G. (1977) Diet and the heart: a postcript. *British Medical Journal*, ii, 1307–1314.

Mott, T. & Roberts, J. (1979) Obesity and hypnosis — a review of the literature. *American Journal of Clinical Hypnosis*, 22, 3–7.

Mrosovsky, N. & Powley, T. L. (1977) Set points for body weight and fat. *Behavioral Biology*, 20, 205–223.

Munro, J. F. (1979) Clinical aspects of the treatment of obesity by drugs: a review. *International Journal of Obesity*, 3, 171–180.

Munro, J. F., MacCuish, A. C., Wilson, E. M. & Duncan, L. J. P. (1968) Comparison of continuous and intermittent anorectic therapy in obesity. *British Medical Journal* i, 352–354.

Munro, H. N. (1964) The significance of labile reserves of body protein. In *Requirements of man for protein*, Ministry of Health Report III, pp 57–62, HMSO, London.

Naeye, R. L. (1979) Weight gain and the outcome of pregnancy. *American Journal of Obstetrics and Gynecology*, **135**, 3–9.

National Academy of Sciences and National Research Council (1964) *Recommended dietary allowances*, 6th revised edition. Food and Nutrition Board, Washington, D.C.

Neel, J. V. (1962) Diabetes mellitus: a 'thrifty' genotype rendered detrimental by 'progress'? *American Journal of Human Genetics*, **14**, 353–362.

Newens, E. M. & Goldstein, H. (1972) Height, weight, and the assessment of obesity in children. *British Journal of Preventive and Social Medicine*, **26**, 33–39.

Nishizawa, T., Akaoka, I., Nishida, Y., Kawaguchi, Y., Hayashi, E. & Yoshimura, T. (1976) Some factors related to obesity in the Japanese sumo wrestler. *American Journal of Clinical Nutrition*, **29**, 1167–1174.

Norgan, N. G. & Durnin, J. V. G. A. (1980) The effect of 6 weeks overfeeding on the body weight, body composition, and energy metabolism of young men. *American Journal of Clinical Nutrition*, **33**, 978–988.

Oliver, M. F. (1978) Diet and coronary heart disease. In *Diet of man: needs and wants*, ed. Yudkin, J., pp. 69–88. London: Applied Science Publishers.

Olsson, K-E. & Saltin, B. (1970) Variation in total body water with muscle glycogen in man. *Acta Physiologica Scandinavica*, **80**, 11–18.

O'Neil, P. M., Currey, H. S., Hirsch, A. A., Riddle, F. E., Taylor, C. I., Malcolm, R. J. & Sexauer, J. D. (1979) Effects of sex of subject and spouse involvement on weightloss in a behavioural treatment program: a retrospective investigation. *Addictive Behaviour*, **4**, 167–177.

Orbach, S. (1978) *Fat is a feminist issue*, p. 192. London, Hamlyn.

Öst, L. G. & Götestam, K. G. (1976) Behavioral and pharmacological treatments for obesity: An experimental comparison. *Addictive Behaviour*, **1**, 331–338.

Pace, N. & Rathbun, E. N. (1945) Studies on body composition: water and chemically combined nitrogen content in relation to fat content. *Journal of Biological Chemistry*, **158**, 685–691.

Parnell, R. W. (1977) How dangerous is obesity? *British Medical Journal*, **i**, 1345–1346.

Passmore, R. & Durnin, J. V. G. A. (1955) Human energy expenditure. *Physiological Reviews*, **35**, 801–840.

Passmore, R., Strong, J. A. & Ritchie, F. J. (1958) The chemical composition of the tissue lost by obese patients on a reducing regimen. *British Journal of Nutrition*, **12**, 113–122.

Paul, A. A. & Southgate, D. A. T. (1978) *McCance and Widdowson's The Composition of Foods*, 4th edition. Ministry of Agriculture, Fisheries and Food and Medical Research Council, HMSO, London.

Peckham, C. H. & Christianson, R. E. (1971) The relationship between pre-pregnancy weight and certain obstetric factors. *American Journal of Obstetrics and Gynecology*, **111**, 1–7.

Penick, S. B., Filion, R., Fox, S. & Stunkard, A. J. (1971) Behavioral modification in the treatment of obesity. *Psychosomatic Medicine*, **33**, 49–55.

Pilkington, T. R. E., Gazet, J. C., Ang, L., Kalucy, R. S., Crisp, A. H. & Day, S. (1976) Explanation for weight loss after ileojejunal bypass in gross obesity. *British Medical Journal*, **i**, 1504–1505.

Pipe, N. G. J., Smith, T., Halliday, D., Edmonds, C. J., Williams, C. & Coltart, T. M. (1979) Changes in fat, fat-free mass and body water in normal human pregnancy. *British Journal of Obstetrics and Gynaecology*, **86**, 929–940.

Pittet, Ph., Chappuis, Ph., Acheson, K., de Techtermann, F. & Jequier, E. (1976) Thermic effect of glucose in obese subjects studied by direct and indirect calorimetry. *British Journal oof Nutrition*, **35**, 281–292.

Pond, D. A. (1979) The training of psychotherapists. *Journal of the Royal Society of Medicine*, **72**, 883–885.

Porikos, K. P., Booth, G. & van Itallie, T. B. (1977) Effect of covert nutritive dilution on the spontaneous food intake of obese individuals: a pilot study. *American Journal of Clinical Nutrition*, **30**, 1638–1644.

Poskitt, E. M. E. & Cole, T. J. (1977) Do fat babies stay fat? *British Medical Journal*, **i**, 7–9.

Prentice, A. M., Whitehead, R. G., Roberts, S., Paul, A., Watkinson, M., Prentice, A. & Watkinson, A. (1980) Dietary supplementation of Gambian nursing mothers and lactational performance. *Lancet*, **ii**, 886–888.

Pudel, V. E. & Oetting, M. (1977) Eating in the laboratory: behavioural aspects of the positive energy balance. *International Journal of Obesity*, **1**, 369–386.

Quetelet, L. A. J. (1871) *Anthropométrie ou mesure des différentes facultés de l'homme*. p. 479. C. Muquardt, Brussels.

Rabast, U., Kasper, H. & Schöborn, J. (1978) Comparative studies in obese subjects fed carbohydrate-restricted and high-carbohydrate 1000-calorie formula diets. *Nutrition Metabolism*, **22**, 269–277.

Ramsay, L. E., Ramsay, M. H., Hettiarachchi, J., Davies, E. L. & Winchester, J. (1978) Weight reduction in a blood pressure clinic. *British Medical Journal*, **ii**, 244–245.

Rand, C. & Stunkard, A. J. (1978) Obesity and psychoanalysis *American Journal of Psychiatry*, **135**, 547–551.

Reed, R. B. & Burke, B. S. (1954) Collection and analysis of dietary intake data. *American Journal of Public Health*, **44**, 1015–1026.

Reuben, D. (1975) *The save your life diet*, Ebury Press, London.

Rimm, I. J. & Rimm, A. A. (1976) Association between juvenile onset obesity and severe adult obesity in 73,532 women. *American Journal of Public Health*, **66**, 479–481.

Rimm, A., Werner, L. H., Van Yserloo, B. & Bernstein, R. A. (1975) Relationship of obesity to disease in 73,522 weight-conscious women. *Public Health Reports*, **90**, 44–52.

Ringrose, C. A. D. (1979) The use of hypnosis as an adjunct to curb obesity. *Public Health*, **93**, 252–257.

Ritt, R. S., Jordan, H. A. & Levitz, L. S. (1979) Changes in nutrient intake a behavioral weight control program. *Journal of the American Dietetic Association*, **74**, 325–330.

Robbins, T. W. & Fray, P. J. (1980) Stress-induced eating: fact, fiction or misunderstanding? *Appetite*, **1**, 103–133.

Robinson, R. G., Folstein, M. F. & McHugh, P. R. (1979) Reduced caloric intake following small bowel bypass surgery: a systematic study of possible causes. *Psychological Medicine*, **9**, 37–53.

Rodin, J. (1980) Changes in perceptual responsiveness following jejunoileostomy: their potential role in reducing food intake. *American Journal of Clinical Nutrition*, **33**, 457–464.

Rodin, J., Bray, G. A., Atkinson, R. L., Dahms, W. T., Greenway, F. L., Hamilton, K. & Molitch, M. (1977) Predictors of successful weight loss in an outpatient obesity clinic. *International Journal of Obesity*, **1**, 79–87.

Rodgers, S., Burnet, R., Goss, A., Phillips, P., Goldney, R., Kimber, C., Thomas, D., Harding, P. & Wise, P. (1977) Jaw wiring in the treatment of obesity. *Lancet*, **i**, 1221–1223.

Rolls, B. J., Rolls, E. T. & Rowe, E. A. (1979) Sensory specific satiety and appetite. *International Journal of Obesity*, **3**, 397–398.

Rothwell, N. J. & Stock, M. J. (1979) A role for brown adipose tissue in diet-induced thermogenesis. *Nature*, **281**, 31–35.

Rudinger, E. (1978) *Which? way to slim*. p. 205. London, Consumers' Association.

Russek, M. (1976) A conceptual equation of intake control. In *Hunger: Basic Mechanisms and Clinical Implications*, ed. Novin, D., Wyrwicka, W. & Bray, G. pp. 327–347. Raven Press, New York.

Salans, L. B., Bray, G. A., Cushman, S. W., Danforth, E. jr., Glennon, J. A., Horton, E. S. & Sims, E. A. H. (1974) Glucose metabolism and the response to insulin by human adipose tissue in spontaneous and experimental obesity. *Journal of Clinical Investigation,* **53,** 848–856.

Sands, J., Dobbing, J. & Gratrix, C. A. (1979) Cell number and cell size: organ growth and development and the control of catch-up growth in rats. *Lancet,* **ii,** 503–505.

Santesson, J. & Nordentröm, J. (1978) Pulmonary function in extreme obesity. Influence of weight loss following intestinal shunt operation. *Acta Chirurgica Scandinavica Supplements* **482,** 36–40.

Sauberlich, H. E., Herman, Y. F., Stevens, C. O. & Herman, R. H. (1979) Thiamin requirement of the human adult. *American Journal of Clinical Nutrition,* **32,** 2237–2248.

Schachter, S. (1968) Obesity and eating: internal and external cues differentially affect the eating behaviour of obese and normal subjects. *Science,* **161,** 751–856.

Sclafani, A. (1978) Dietary obesity. In *Recent Advances in Obesity Research: 2,* ed. Bray, G., pp. 123–132. Newman Publishing. London.

Scopinaro, N., Gianetta, E., Civalleri, D., Bonalumi, U. & Bachi, V. (1980) Two years of experience with bilio-pancreatic bypass for obesity. *American Journal of Clinical Nutrition,* **33,** 506–514.

Scorbie, I. N., Durward, W. F. & MacCuish, A. C. (1980) Proximal myopathy after prolonged total therapeutic starvation. *British Medical Journal,* **280,** 1212–1213.

Scrignar, C. B. (1980) Mandatory weight control program for 550 police officers choosing either behavior modification or 'willpower'. *Obesity and Bariatric Medicine,* **9,** 88–92.

Seaton, D. A. & Rose, K. (1965) Defaulters from a weight reduction clinic. *Journal of Chronic Diseases,* **18,** 1007–1011.

Sebrell, W. H. (1975) The nutritional adequacy of reducing diets. In *Recent advances in obesity research: 1,* ed. Howard, A., pp. 286–288, London: Newman Publishing.

Seddon, R., Penfound, J. & Garrow, J. S. (1981) The Harrow Slimming Club: Analysis of the results obtained in 249 members of a self-financing, non-profit-making group. *Journal of Human Nutrition.*

Sedgewick, A. W., Brotherhood, J. R., Harris-Davidson, A., Taplin, R. & Thomas, D. W. (1980) Long-term effects of physical training programme on risk factors for coronary heart disease in otherwise sedentary men. *British Medical Journal,* **281,** 7–10.

Seltzer, C. C. (1966) Some re-evaluations of the build and blood pressure study 1959 as related to ponderal index, somatotype and mortality. *New England Journal of Medicine,* **274,** 254–259.

Seltzer, C. C. & Mayer, J. (1965) A simple criterion of obesity. *Postgraduate Medicine,* **38,** 101–107.

Silverstone, J. T., Stark, J. E. & Buckle, R. M. (1966) Hunger during total starvation. *Lancet,* **i,** 1343–1344.

Simpson, R. W., Mann, J. I., Eaton, J., Moore, R. A., Carter, R. & Hockaday, T. D. R. (1979) Improved glucose control in maturity-onset diabetes treated with a high-carbohydrate modified-fat diet. *British Medical Journal,* **i,** 1753–1756.

Sims, E. A. H., Danforth, E. Jr., Horton, E. S., Bray, G. A., Glennon, J. A. & Salans, L. B. (1973) Endocrine and metabolic effects of experimental obesity in man. *Recent Progress in Hormone Research,* **29,** 457–476.

Sims, E. A. H., Goldman, R. F., Gluck, C. M., Horton, E. S., Kelleher, P. C. & Rowe, D. W. (1968) Experimental obesity in man. *Transactions of the Association of American Physicians,* **81,** 153–170.

Smith, T., Hesp, R. & MacKenzie, J. (1979) Total body potassium calibrations for normal and obese subjects in two types of whole body counter. *Physics in Medicine and Biology,* **24,** 171–175.

Sohar, E., Scapa, E. & Ravid, M. (1973) Constancy of relative body weight in children. *Archives of Disease in Childhood*, **48**, 389–392.

Solow, C., Silberfarb, P. M. & Swift, K. (1974) Psychosocial effects of intestinal bypass surgery for severe obesity. *New England Journal of Medicine*, **290**, 300–304.

Sorlie, P., Gordon, T. & Kannel, W. B. (1980) Body build and mortality: the Framingham study. *Journal of the American Medical Association*, **243**, 1828–1831.

Southgate, D. A. T. (1976) The definition and analysis of dietary fibre. In *Food and fibre*, Marabou Symposium, Sundbyberg.

Southgate, D. A. T., Bingham, S. & Robertson, J. (1978) Dietary fibre in the British diet. *Nature*, **247**, 51–52.

Spiegel, T. A. (1973) Caloric regulation of food intake in man. *Journal of Comparative and Physiological Psychology*, **84**, 24–37.

Spinnler, G., Jéquier, E., Fabre, R., Dolivo, M. & Vanotti, A. (1973) Human calorimeter with a new type of gradient layer. *Journal of Applied Physiology*, **35**, 158–165.

Stamler, J. Farino, E., Mojonnier, L. M., Hall, Y., Moss, D. & Stamler, R. (1980) Prevention and control of hypertension by nutritional-hygeinic means. *Journal of the American Medical Association*, **243**, 1819–1823.

Stanton, H. E. (1975) Weight loss through hypnosis. *American Journal of ClinicalHypnosis*, **18**, 94–97.

Stanton, H. E. (1976) Fee-paying and weight loss: evidence for an interesting interaction. *American Journal of Clinical Hypnosis*, **19**, 47–49.

Steel, J. M. & Briggs, M. (1972) Withdrawal depression in obese patients after fenfluramine treatment. *British Medical Journal*, iii, 26–27.

Steel, J. M., Munro, J. F. & Duncan, L. J. P. (1973) A comparative trial of different regimens of fenfluramine and phentermine in obesity. *Practitioner*, **211**, 232–236.

Stein, Z., Susser, M., Saenger, G. & Marolla, F. (1975) *Famine and Human Development: the Dutch winter hunger of 1944–1945.* p. 284. New York, Oxford University Press.

Stock, M. (1981) Thermogenic response to overfeeding lean animals. In *Recent advances in obesity research: 3*, eds. Howard, A. N., Björntorp, P. & Cairella, M. London: John Libbey.

Stock, A. L. & Yudkin, J. (1970) Nutrient intake of subjects on a low carbohydrate diet used in treatment of obesity. *American Journal of Clinical Nutrition*, **23**, 948–952.

Storr, A. (1979) *The Art of Psychotherapy*, pp. 191, Secker & Warburg, London.

Strain, G. W. & Strain, J. J. (1979) Psychological impediments to weight loss. *International Journal of Obesity*, **3**, 167–170

Strata. A., Ugolotti, G., Contini, C., Magnati, G., Pugnoli, C., Tirelli, F. & Zuliani, U. (1978) Thyroid and obesity: survey of some function tests in a large obese population. *International Journal of Obesity*, **2**, 333–340.

Strauss, R. J. & Wise, L. (1978) Operative risks of obesity. *Surgery, Gynecology and Obstetrics*, **146**, 286–291.

Stuart, R. B. (1967) Behavioural control of overeating. *Behaviour Research and Therapy*, **5**, 357–365.

Stunkard, A. J. (1972) New therapies for the eating disorders: Behaviour modification of obesity and anorexia nervosa. *Archives of General Psychiatry*, **26**, 391–398.

Stunkard, A. J. (1975) Obesity and social environment. In *Recent Advances in obesity research: I*, ed. Howard, A., pp. 178–190. London: Newman Publishing.

Stunkard, A. J. (1978) The development of tolerance to appetite suppressant medication: new theory, new hope. *Journal of Psychedelic Drugs*, **10**, 331–341.

Stunkard, A. J. & Brownell, K. D. (1980) Work-site treatment for obesity. *American Journal of Psychiatry*, **137**, 252–253.

Stunkard, A. J., Craighead, L. W. & O'Brien, R. (1980) Controlled trial of behaviour therapy, pharmacotherapy, and their combination in the treatment of obesity. *Lancet,* **ii,** 1045–1047.

Stunkard, A. & Kaplan, D. (1977) Eating in public places: A review of reports of direct observation of eating behaviour. *International Journal of Obesity,* **1,** 89–101.

Stunkard, A. J. & Penick, S. B. (1979) Behavior modification in the treatment of obesity. *Archives of General Psychiatry,* **36,** 801–806.

Sullivan, A. C. & Comai, K. (1978) Pharmacological treatment of obesity. *International Journal of Obesity,* **2,** 167–189.

Sullivan, L. (1976) Metabolic and physiologic effects of physical training in hyperplastic obesity. *Scandinavian Journal of Rehabilitation Medicine,* **suppl. 5,** p. 38.

Sveger, T. (1978) Does overnutrition or obesity during the first year affect weight at age four? *Acta Paediatrica Scandinavica,* **67,** 465–468.

Taylor, H. L., Jacobs, D. R., Schucker, B., Knudsen, J., Leon, A. S. & Debacker, G. (1978) A questionnaire for the assessment of leisure time physical activities. *Journal of Chronic Diseases,* **31,** 741–745.

Tilker, H. & Meyer, R. (1972) The use of covert sensitisation and hypnotic procedures in the treatment of the overweight person: a case report. *American Journal of Clinical Hypnosis,* **15,** 15–19.

Truswell, A. S. (1978) Minimal estimates of needs and recommended intakes of nutrients. In *Diet of Man: needs and wants,* ed. Yudkin, J., pp. 5–24. London, Applied Science Publication.

Tschegg, E., Sigmund, A., Veitl, V., Schmid, P. & Irsigler, K. (1979) An isothermic, gradient-free, whole body calorimeter for long-term investigations of energy balance in man. *Metabolism,* **28,** 764–770.

Tullis, I. F. (1973) Rational diet for mild and grand obesity. *Journal of the American Medical Association,* **226,** 70–73.

Turner, P. (1978) How do anti-obesity drugs work? *International Journal of Obesity,* **2,** 343–348.

Udall, J. N., Garrison, G. G., Vaucher, Y., Walson, P. D. & Morrow, G. (1978) Interaction of maternal and neonatal obesity. *Pediatrics,* **62,** 17–21.

U.S. Department of Health, Education and Welfare (1979) *Dietary intake source data, United States 1971–74.* National Center for Health Statistics, Maryland.

U.S. Senate Select Committee on Nutrition and Human Needs (1977) *Dietary goals for the United States,* Washington, D.C.: U.S. Government Printing Office.

Vagenakis, A. G., Burger, A., Portnay, G. I., Rudolph, M., O'Brian, J. T., Azizi, F., Arky, R. A., Nicod, P., Ingbar, S. H. & Braverman, L. E. (1975) Diversion of peripheral thyroxine metabolism from activating to inactivating pathways during complete fasting. *Journal of Clinical Endocrinology and Metabolism,* **41,** 191–194.

van Itallie, T. B. (1978) Dietary fibre and obesity., *American Journal of Clinical Nutrition,* **31** (10 suppl), S43–52.

van Itallie, T. B. & Yang, M-U (1977) Nitrogen balance during weight reduction: effect of body stores of protein and fat. In *Recent advances in obesity research: 2,* ed. Bray, G., pp. 379–384. London: Newman Publishing

van Stratum, P., Lussenburg, R. N., van Wezel, L. A., Vergroesen, A. J. & Cremer, H. D. (1978) The effect of dietary carbohydrate:fat ratio on energy intake by adult women. *American Journal of Clinical Nutrition,* **31,** 206–212.

Vertes, V., Genuth, S. M. & Hazleton, I. M. (1977a) Precautions with supplemented fasting. *Journal of the American Medical Association,* **238,** 2142.

Vertes, V., Genuth, S. M. & Hazelton, I. M. (1977b) Supplemented fasting as a large-scale out patient program. *Journal of the American Medical Association,* **238,** 2151–2153.

Vignati, L., Finley, R. J., Hagg, S. & Aoki, T. T. (1978) Protein conservation during prolonged fast: a function of triiodothyronine levels. *Transactions of the Association of American Physicians,* **91,** 169–179.

Villar, H. V., Burks, T. F. & Wangenstein, S. L. (1979) Mechanisms of satiety after gastric stapling and gastric bypass. *Surgical Forum*, 30, 353-355.

Voit, C. (1866) uber die Verschiedenheiten der Eiweiss zersetzung beim Hungern. *Zeitschrift für Biologie*, 2, 307-365.

Wales, J. K. (1980) The effect of fenfluramine on weight loss during restricted dietary regimes. *International Journal of Obesity*, 4, 127-132.

Warnold, I. & Lenner, R. A. (1977) Evaluation of the heart rate method to determine the daily energy expenditure in disease. A study on juvenile diabetics. *American Journal of Clinical Nutrition*, 30, 304-315.

Warwick, P. M. & Garrow, J. S. (1981) The effect of addition of exercise to a regime of dietary restriction on weight loss, nitrogen balance, resting metabolic rate and spontaneous physical activity in three obese women in a metabolic ward. *International Journal of Obesity*, 5.

Warwick, P. M., Toft, R. & Garrow, J. S. (1978) Individual variation in energy expenditure. *International Journal of Obesity*, 2, 396.

Waxman, M. & Stunkard, A. J. (1980) Caloric intake and expenditure of obese boys. *Journal of Pediatrics*, 96, 187-193.

Webb, P., Annis, J. F. & Troutman, S. J. (1972) Human calorimetry with a water-cooled garment. *Journal of Applied Physiology*, 32, 412-418.

Weiner, M. F. (1980) Rapid weight gain due to overinsulinization. *Obesity and Bariatric Medicine*, 9, 118-119.

Weisenberg, M. & Frey, E. (1974) What's missing in the treatment of obesity by behaviour modification? *Journal of the American Dietetic Association*, 65, 410-414.

West, K. M. (1980) Computing and expressing degrees of fatness. *Journal of the American Medical Association*, 243, 1421-1422.

Whitelaw, A. G. L. (1976) Influence of maternal obesity on subcutaneous fat in the newborn. *British Medical Journal*, i, 985-986.

Widdowson, E. M. (1936) A study of English diets by the individual method. Part I. Men. *Journal of Hygiene (London)*, 36, 269-292.

Widdowson, E. M. (1951) Studies in undernutrition, Wuppertal 1946-49. The response to unlimited food. *Medical Research Council Special Report Series*, No. 275, 313-344. London, H.M.S.O.

Widdowson, E. M. (1962) Nutritional individuality. *Proceedings of the Nutrition Society*, 21, 121-128.

Widdowson, E. M. & Dickerson, J. W. T. (1960) The effect of growth and function on the chemical composition of soft tissues. *Biochemical Journal*, 77, 30-43.

Widdowson, E. M., Edholm, O. G. & McCance, R. A. (1954) The food intake and energy expenditure of cadets in training. *British Journal of Nutrition*, 8, 147-155.

Widdowson, E. M., McCance, R. A. & Spray, C. M. (1951) The chemical composition of the human body. *Clinical Science*, 10, 113-125.

Wilkinson, L. H. (1980) Reduction of gastric reservoir capacity. *American Journal of Clinical Nutrition*, 33, 515-517.

Wilkinson, P. W., Parkin, J. M., Pearlson, J., Philips, P. R. & Sykes, P. (1977) Obesity in childhood: a community study in Newcastle upon Tyne. *Lancet*, i, 350-352.

Wilmore, J. H., Brown, C. H. & Davis, J. A. (1977) Body physique and composition of the female distance runner. *Annals of the New York Academy of Sciences*, 301, 764-776.

Wilson, E. A., Hadden, D. R., Merrett, J. D., Montgomery, D. A. D. & Weaver, J. A.(1980) Dietary management of maturity onset diabetes. *British Medical Journal*, 280, 1367-1369.

Wilson, G. T. & Brownell, K. D. (1978) Behavior therapy for obesity: including family members in the treatment process. *Behavior Therapy*, 9, 943-945.

Wilson, J. H. P. & Lamberts, S. W. J. (1979) Nitrogen balance in obese patients receiving a very low calorie liquid formula diet. *American Journal of Clinical Nutrition*, 32, 1612-1616.

Wing, R. R. & Jeffery, R. W. (1979) Outpatient treatments of obesity: a comparison of methodology and clinical results. *International Journal of Obesity*, 3, 261–279.

Winick, M. (1979) ed. *Hunger disease*, pp. 261, New York, John Wiley.

Winkelstein, L. B. (1959) Hypnosis, diet and weight reduction. *New York State Journal of Medicine*, 59, 1751–1756.

Womersley, J. & Durnin, J. V. G. A. (1977) A comparison of the skinfold method with extent of 'overweight' and various weight-height relationships in the assessment of obesity. *British Journal of Nutrition*, 38, 271–284.

Wood, G. D. (1977) Early results of treatment of the obese by a diet regimen enforced by maxillomandibular fixation. *Journal of Oral Surgery*, 35, 461–363.

Wooley, O. W. (1971) Long-term food regulation in the obese and non-obese. *Psychosomatic Medicine*, 33, 436–444.

Wooley, O. W., Wooley, S. C. & Dunham, R. B. (1972) Can calories be perceived, and do they affect hunger in obese and non-obese humans? *Journal of Comparative and Physiological Psychology*, 80, 250–258.

Wooley, S. C., Wooley, O. W. & Dyrenforth, S. (1980) The case against radical interventions. *American Journal of Clinical Nutrition*, 33, 465–471.

Yang, M. U. & van Itallie, T. B. (1976) Composition of weight loss during short-term weight reduction. *Journal of Clinical Investigation*, 58, 722–730.

Yates, B. T. (1980) Survey comparison of success, morbidity, mortality, fees and psychological benefits and costs of 3,146 patients receiving jejunoileal or gastric bypass. *American Journal of Clinical Nutrition*, 33, 518–522.

Yudkin, J. (1958) *This slimming business*. London: MacGibbon & Kee.

Yudkin, J. (1963) Nutrition and palatability with special reference to obesity, myocardial infarction, and other diseases of civilization. *Lancet*, i, 1335–1338.

Yudkin, J. (1974) The low-carbohydrate diet, in: *Obesity*, ed. Burland, W. L., Samuel, P. D. & Yudkin, J. pp. 271–280. Edinburgh, Churchill Livingstone.

Zack, F. M., Harlan, W. R., Leaverton, P. E. & Cornoni-Huntley, J. (1979) A longitudinal study of body fatness in childhood and adolescence. *Journal of Pediatrics*, 95, 126–130.

Zuti, W. B. & Golding, L. A. (1976) Comparing diet and exercise as weight reduction tools. *Physician and Sportsmedicine*, 4, 49–53.

Author Index

Subject index

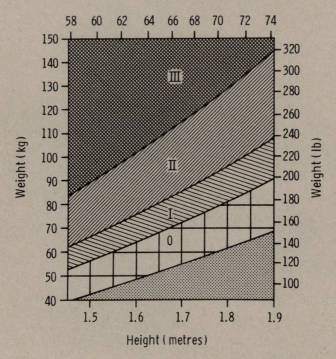

Fig. 1.3 Relation of weight to height defining the desirable range (0), and grades I, II and III obesity, marked by the boundaries W/H^2 = 25–29.9, 30–40, and over 40 respectively (*see also* page 6)